Dedication

"Dedicated to Frances M. Myrick, a wonderful
human being and mother."
— *Florence*

"Dedicated in memory to Martin Yonge, always
supportive and reflective."
— *Olive*

Special Dedication
To those nurses who in their roles as preceptors
so willingly give of their time, expertise, and
wisdom in preparing the future nurses of this
great profession.

Nursing Preceptorship

CONNECTING PRACTICE AND EDUCATION

Nursing Preceptorship

CONNECTING PRACTICE AND EDUCATION

Florence Myrick, RN, BN, MScN, PhD
Associate Professor
University of Alberta
Edmonton, Alberta
Canada

Olive Yonge, RN, MEd, PhD, CPsych
Professor
University of Alberta
Edmonton, Alberta
Canada

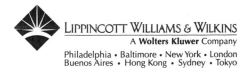

LIPPINCOTT WILLIAMS & WILKINS
A **Wolters Kluwer** Company
Philadelphia • Baltimore • New York • London
Buenos Aires • Hong Kong • Sydney • Tokyo

Senior Acquisitions Editor: Patricia Casey
Editorial Assistant: Dana Irwin
Production Editor: Danielle Michaely
Director of Nursing Production: Helen Ewan
Design Coordinator: Brett MacNaughton

Manufacturing Manager: William Alberti
Indexer: Angie Wiley
Compositor: Lippincott Williams & Wilkins
Printer: R.R. Donnelley-Crawfordsville

9 8 7 6 5 4 3 2 1

Library of Congress Cataloging-in-Publication Data

Myrick, Florence.
   Nursing preceptorship : connecting practice and education / Florence Myrick,
   Olive Yonge.
     p. ; cm
   Includes bibliographical references and index.
   ISBN 0-7817-5065-2 (alk. paper)
   1. Nursing--Study and teaching (Preceptorship) I. Yonge, Olive. II Title.
   [DNLM: 1. Education, Nursing, Baccalaureate. 2. Preceptorship. WY 18.5 M998n 2004]
   RT74.7.M97 2004
   610.73'071--dc22

                            2003065927

Care has been taken to confirm the accuracy of the information presented and to describe generally accepted practices. However, the
authors, editors, and publisher are not responsible for errors or omis-
sions or for any consequences from application of the information in
this book and make no warranty, express or implied, with respect to the
content of the publication.

The authors, editors, and publisher have exerted every effort to ensure
that drug selection and dosage set forth in this text are in accordance
with the current recommendations and practice at the time of publication. However, in view of ongoing research, changes in government regulations, and the constant flow of information relating to drug therapy
and drug reactions, the reader is urged to check the package insert for
each drug for any change in indications and dosage and for added warn-
ings and precautions. This is particularly important when the recommended agent is a new or infrequently employed drug.
Some drugs and medical devices presented in this publication have
Food and Drug Administration (FDA) clearance for limited use in
restricted research settings. It is the responsibility of the health care
provider to ascertain the FDA status of each drug or device planned for
use in his or her clinical practice.

LWW.com

Reviewers

Judith Boone, MSN, RN
Nurse Manager
Salem Hospital, North Shore Medical Center
Salem, Massachusetts

Sue Chambers, RNC, BSN
Perinatal Director
Fremont Medical Center
Yuba City, California

Andrew G. Escamilla, MS, RN
CEO
Kindred Hospital Boston North Shore
Peabody, Massachusetts

Kathleen Kirby, RN
Program Coordinator
Rural California Nursing Preceptorship Program
California State University, Chico
Chico, California

Patricia Melanson, MN, RN
Associate Professor
Dalhousie University School of Nursing
Halifax, Nova Scotia
Canada

Judith Scanlan, RN, PhD
Associate Professor
Faculty of Nursing
University of Manitoba
Winnipeg, Manitoba

Rick Vanderlee, RN, BNSc, MScN, EdD
Director, Learning and Development
Calgary Health Region
Calgary, Alberta

Introduction

The world of nursing is fast becoming increasingly complex. Nowhere is that more apparent than with the practicing nurse who must assume a diverse array of roles and responsibilities, not the least of which encompasses that of preceptor with all of its own intrinsic complexities. Daily, preceptors must prepare graduates who are "adept at coping with the growing body of nursing knowledge, the rapid advances in science and technology, and the economic constraints that continue to result in massive health care changes" (Myrick, 2002, p. 154). They are confronted daily with the challenge of preparing clinically competent practitioners who must not only survive, but also thrive in an ever-changing and always multifaceted system. It is, therefore, incumbent on those within the nursing profession to provide nurses who assume the preceptor role with appropriate support mechanisms that will facilitate them in their endeavor. This book offers a dimension of that support, the purpose of which is threefold: 1) to provide practicing nurses with a framework and conceptual resource for their role in the preceptorship experience; 2) to augment ongoing workshops for staff nurse preceptors; and 3) to supplement course materials in clinical or practicum courses in which preceptorship is utilized for student learning in the practice setting.

While the primary goal of this book is to facilitate the preceptorship experience for nurse preceptors, secondarily, it will also provide a framework or resource for students, faculty, staff, and others who are involved in the preceptorship experience. As well, owing to its substantive nature, this book can be utilized quite readily by other professional disciplines in which the field or practicum experience assumes a central focus in their academic programs.

Over the years, preceptorship has fast become the leading approach to clinical teaching in undergraduate nursing programs in Australia, Canada, the United Kingdom, and the United States (Usher, Nolan, Reser, Owens, & Tollefson, 1999). Preceptorship has come to be recognized as the approach of choice for orienting new graduates and staff nurses to the practice setting (Hardyman & Hickey, 2001). At a recent conference in Copenhagen, Denmark (June 2001), attended by over 4,000 nurses from 120 countries worldwide, the interest in preceptorship was noticeably widespread. It is important, therefore, that every effort be made to strengthen the preceptorship approach to clinical teaching because in doing so, not only is the preparation of our future practitioners assured but the profession of nursing itself and the society that it serves will be the ultimate beneficiaries.

Being responsible for the teaching of the future practitioners of the nursing profession is no easy achievement. It is sometimes a daunting but always a rewarding proposition. It is particularly so when those who are expected to assume that responsibility often possess minimal or no formal preparation to take on that challenge, which is why the authors believe this book will be of considerable assistance to those nurses who assume such a critical role. How best can appropriate and ongoing support be provided to facilitate preceptors in fulfilling the responsibility that has been thrust upon them? While, over the years, orientation programs have been developed and implemented to support nurses in their preceptor endeavor, it is not an uncommon occurrence for such programs to dissolve within a short period of time. The dissolution of such programs is often related to widespread nursing shortages and the ongoing inability of administrators to free up the nurses' time for attending such sessions. A book such as this one can fill a huge gap that is evident in the preparation and ongoing support of the preceptor. As well, it can fill a void by providing a resource to faculty, students, and staff by clearly delineating the kinds of roles and responsibilities that they assume in the preceptorship experience.

The reader may pose the question as to the real benefits of a model such as preceptorship. When examined
closely, it becomes apparent that this approach to clinical teaching impacts the profession on two levels. The
first is on a macro or big picture level, and the second is
on a micro level. The authors would posit that it is
because of the preceptorship approach to clinical teaching that the nursing worlds of practice and education
have coalesced in a collaborative way. Within this context, practicing nurses connect daily with nursing faculty to create a hospitable climate, one that is supportive of the teaching-learning process, and in doing so
share their diverse perspectives to help shape the
preparation of future practitioners and leaders of the
profession.

In Chapter One, the authors discuss the different
dimensions of the preceptorship experience. They
address the emergence of preceptorship on the nursing
landscape and the critical role that it has come to play
within the profession. Preceptorship requires a delicate
balance between the domains of practice and education,
and when implemented appropriately, it can serve to
strengthen what at times has become a tenuous
alliance. The authors discuss procedures that can be
instituted to facilitate this process. Effective communication, routine visitations, regular faculty contact with
the clinical units on which students are assigned, and a
formalized process of faculty-preceptor interaction are
some practices that can contribute to the creation of a
collaborative process that lends strength to the linkages
between practice and education. Collaborative relationships are discussed, with a special emphasis on the
importance of the practice setting's contribution to the
creation of a climate that is supportive of the education
of nursing students.

Chapter Two addresses directly the teaching-learning
climate to be established in the preceptorship experience. Discussion is derived from research revealing the
notion that for student learning to be maximized to its
full potential, the climate in which students are
assigned must be one in which they feel a sense of
safety, respect, and acceptance as beginning practition-

ers (Myrick & Yonge, 2002). The creation of such a climate is not only the responsibility of the preceptor and the staff on the particular nursing units, but also must be reflective of the ongoing involvement of nursing faculty. All too often faculty members assume a peripheral role with regard to the preceptorship experience. At times they even seem at arm's length or marginalized. Frequently, such minimal participation can not only result in negative fallout for student learning, progress, and evaluation, but can also precipitate unnecessary tension between the preceptor and the faculty members, thus straining an already fragile liaison. In other words, it should not be an expectation of the preceptorship experience that preceptors alone assume complete responsibility for student learning. It is essential that faculty assume an active role in partnership with the preceptor. Discussion explores key issues within this context.

Chapter Three focuses specifically on the major players in the preceptorship experience: those in clinical practice—the preceptor and the staff—and those in education, in particular the preceptee and the faculty. This chapter is devoted to a detailed discussion of the roles of each of the key players and a delineation of their respective responsibilities. Discussion is derived from research in the area of preceptorship and the works of various scholars in this area, including the authors themselves (Myrick & Yonge, 2002; Yonge, Myrick, & Haase, 2002). Role model, teacher, facilitator, guide, evaluator, and guardian will be identified as the major roles assumed by the preceptor and originate directly from recent research (Myrick, 2002). Each of these roles is discussed at length and suggestions are proposed as to how the preceptor can effectively address these within the context of the practice setting.

While the involvement of the staff is assumed to be somewhat marginal to the preceptorship experience, the authors posit that staff acceptance of students contributes directly to its success. The relationship between the staff and the preceptor will be addressed also and how it impacts directly on student learning. As well, other roles such as clinical resource and contributor to the evaluation process will be discussed, specifically in relation to staff involvement.

The role of faculty within the context of the preceptorship experience has tended to become somewhat peripheral in nature. While preceptorship was originally intended to include a tripartite arrangement that directly involved the faculty, preceptor, and preceptee, instead, more and more, the preceptorship experience has evolved to include primarily the preceptor/preceptee dyad. In this chapter, the authors discuss how the role of faculty, when appropriately utilized, is integral to the success of the preceptorship experience. The authors suggest that the faculty members must assume key roles in the preceptorship experience that include resource, custodian of the teaching-learning process, and evaluator. As a resource, it is essential that faculty members be available and accessible (Whittaker, Davies, Thompson, & Shepherd, 1997). As custodians of the teaching-learning process and evaluators, it is critical that faculty members ascertain regular feedback about the students' progress and ensure that their experience is congruent with program and learning objectives. Finally, to ensure that the evaluation process is effective, it is also important that faculty provide appropriate guidelines to both preceptor and preceptee with regard to the substantive nature of the learning experience and delineate how best that fits with the process required to accommodate such content. Intrinsic to the evaluator faculty role as well is the necessity for preceptor evaluation. It is essential that faculty members determine how well the preceptor functions as a clinical teacher to the preceptee. Opportunities need to be sought in which faculty member and preceptor can collaborate and discuss how well the preceptor is facilitating the preceptees' learning, and the faculty member can provide constructive feedback on the preceptor's performance in this regard.

The role of the student or preceptee is also addressed. The authors emphasize the students' need to be active participants demonstrating professionalism, reliability, accountability, and responsibility for self-evaluation. Active participation on the part of students and ongoing input are keys to a rewarding experience.

Chapter Four focuses on the goals and objectives of the preceptorship experience and addresses the substantive nature of the teaching-learning experience within the context of preceptorship. There are a number of perspectives, including teachers of the educational programs, administrators of the practice agencies, preceptors, and preceptees. The authors reflect on what should be going on in the preceptorship experience with regard to these different perspectives and show how they converge around the preceptorship experience to ensure a successful outcome for all groups.

Chapter Five discusses the preceptor as teacher. The authors explore ways in which the preceptor can ensure appropriate selection of patient assignments that are conducive to student learning objectives and preceptor expectations. Strategies are discussed to assist the preceptor in promoting critical thinking and student autonomy. Relevant evaluation techniques are addressed that include a variety of tools to assist the preceptor in facilitating the evaluation process.

In Chapter Six the authors discuss the student as learner. They address the significance of student participation in their own learning and how the preceptor can maximize that participation. While it is often the perspective that students, particularly neophytes to the practice setting, need to be directed in what they do, the authors emphasize the importance of recognizing the individual contributions that students can make regardless of their level of experience. In other words, how well students are valued and respected for themselves impacts directly on how well they perform within the contextual reality of the preceptorship experience. Specifically, the authors emphasize the importance of the preceptors' understanding learning and personality styles. An author-generated learning style assessment tool is included to assist preceptors and preceptees to better understand their learning preferences. The tool has been used in numerous preceptorship preparation workshops with great success.

Chapter Seven is concerned directly with learning opportunities and deals with such issues as personality conflicts that can arise among the various players, questionable competence of student or preceptor, the student who does not progress, and unethical behaviors. Recommendations for resolving such issues are directly explored at length.

Chapter Eight addresses the all-important area of communication. One could hypothesize that communication is fundamental to the success of any relationship. Preceptorship is no exception. It is critical that the communication between preceptor and student, faculty and preceptor, faculty and student, and all three and the staff be constructive and proficient. The authors explore various avenues by which such appropriate communication can be maintained throughout the preceptorship experience and address different dimensions of that communication process. Specifically, the authors discuss how to give feedback, different learning and teaching styles, preparing for the preceptorship experience, and ascertaining closure for the preceptorship experience.

The final chapter, Chapter Nine, is an additional bonus in that it provides some useful suggestions with regard to instituting a preceptorship program. Beginning with preceptor selection criteria, this chapter imparts to the reader some dos and don'ts when considering the prospect of developing and implementing a preceptorship program.

The authors hope that you will find this book beneficial to you as a preceptor, preceptee, faculty member, and staff person, or those of you who are involved in the daily lives of the various learners in the practice setting. While it is designed to be reader friendly, this book is nevertheless derived from research and from a variety of sources that we believe contribute to an evidenced-based teaching-learning model for clinical and community practice.

R E F E R E N C E S

Hardyman, R., & Hickey, G. (2001). What do newly-qualified nurses expect from preceptorship? Exploring the perspective of the preceptee. *Nurse Education Today, 21,* 58–64.

Myrick, F. (2002). Preceptorship and critical thinking in baccalaureate nursing education. *Journal of Nursing Education, 41*(4), 154–164.

Myrick, F., & Yonge, O. (2002). Creating a climate for critical thinking in the preceptorship experience. *Nurse Education Today, 21*(6), 461–467.

Myrick, F., & Yonge, O. (2003). Preceptorship: A quintessential compo-
nent of nursing education. In M. H. Oermann & K. T. Heinrich
(Eds.), *Annual Review of Nursing Education* (Vol. 1). New York:
Springer.

Usher, K., Nolan, C., Reser, P., Owens, J., & Tollefson, J. (1999). An
exploration of the preceptor roles: Preceptors' perceptions of benefits, rewards, supports and commitment to the preceptor role. *Journal of Advanced Nursing, 29*(2), 506–514.

Whittaker, K. A., Davies S., Thompson, A. M., & Shepherd, B. (1997). A
survey of community placements for educational programmes in
nursing and midwifery. *Nurse Education Today, 17*(6), 463–472.

Yonge, O., Myrick, F., & Hasse, M. (2002). Student nurse stress in the
preceptorship experience. *Nurse Educator, 27*(2), 84–88.

Contents

PART I

Context

Shaping the Preceptorship Experience

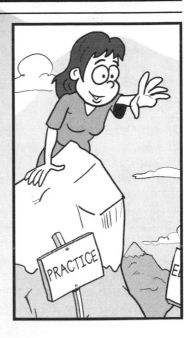

Preceptorship is a model or approach to teaching-learning in the practice or field setting that pairs students or novice nurses with experienced practitioners. Specifically, it is "an individualized teaching-learning method in which each student is assigned to a particular preceptor...so she [or he] experiences day-to-day practice with a role model and resource person immediately available within the clinical setting" (Chickerella & Lutz, 1981). Such pairing intends to foster professional socialization, enhance learning, promote critical thinking, cultivate practical wisdom, and facilitate competence. However, understanding the contextual reality of the preceptorship approach to clinical teaching requires some knowledge of the history of preceptorship. Building on that background, this chapter examines the critical role that the preceptorship experience assumes and where preceptorship fits within the realm of nursing. Preceptorship occupies a strategic space, connecting the domains of practice and education. It provides a collaborative opportunity for practicing nurses and faculty. This chapter addresses the benefits that accrue from this approach to teaching-learning, specifically as they relate to the practice and educational settings and the key players for whom preceptorship has the most direct consequences.

• The Emergence of Preceptorship in Nursing

Preceptorship is not an entirely new concept in the nursing profession. It has been an important dimension of nursing since its origins during the time of Florence Nightingale, when nurses were expected to facilitate student nurses in their learning and to guide them in the care of their patients in the practice setting (Backenstose, 1983; Myrick & Yonge, 2003). During the time of the hospital diploma programs, the concept of preceptorship slipped into obscurity and remained dormant for several decades. However, in the 1960s, preceptorship emerged again as a legitimate approach to clinical teaching, when nurse practitioner programs in the United States resurrected it for teaching students. Thus, preceptorship introduced the formal use of experienced nurses to assist students in meeting specific educational/learning objectives in the practice setting. However, originally physicians were used as preceptors, because it was the belief at the time that nurses lacked the experience and ability to teach. Also, the use of preceptors was a common practice in the medical profession (Backenstose, 1983). In addition to the emergence of preceptorship in nurse practitioner programs, the transfer of nursing education from hospitals to postsecondary institutions at that time contributed to the rise of its prominence. Coinciding with this move was a growing concern that immediately on the acquisition of staff nurse positions, new graduates were unable to assume full patient-care responsibilities in accordance with employer expectations (Myrick & Awrey, 1988). This difficulty in making the transition from student nurse to staff nurse was a phenomenon referred to as "reality shock," a theme that would become all too familiar to both educators and practicing nurses (Kramer, 1974). Since the 1970s, preceptorship has continued to gain momentum. Today, it has become a highly effective approach to the clinical teaching of nursing students and an integral part of the orientation of new nurses in the practice setting (Hardyman & Hickey, 2001; Myrick & Barrett, 1992; Usher, Nolan, Reser, Owens, & Tollefson, 1999). For information on orientating new staff, see Box 1-1.

• Connecting Practice and Education:
A Strategic Space for Preceptorship

During the last several decades, the numerous changes that have occurred in the nursing profession and in the health care field in general have not occurred in isolation. The effect on the content and process of

Box 1-1. Serving as Preceptor to New Staff

Unlike student preceptorship, serving as preceptor to staff does not involve the participation of a faculty member. Usually, the preceptees in this instance are staff members who are new to the profession or new to a practice area. Usually the preceptor provides the orientation, teaching, coaching, support, and evaluation of these staff preceptees. Administration, a staff educator, or other staff members may, in turn, support the preceptor. The focus of this type of preceptorship experience is to ensure that the new staff preceptees become oriented as quickly as possible to their role and assume full responsibility within a short time. The assessment of their performance is based on "how well they are doing and fitting in." If the new staff preceptee is on a probationary contract, the preceptor is responsible for being alert to potential performance issues. Whether the preceptor in this case receives orientation to his or her role depends, to a large extent, on the size of the agency, and he or she may thus have to use the resources at his or her immediate disposal.

nursing education is considerable. In response to these many changes, nursing education has employed varied teaching and learning methods or approaches (Fernald, Staudenmaier, Tressler, Main, O'Brien-Gonzales, & Barley, 2001). One such approach, preceptorship, provides a perfect medium in which practice and education can combine to achieve a common goal—the preparation of present and future practitioners and of leaders of the nursing profession. For the preceptorship experience to succeed, those in the education and practice settings must create and nurture a genuine bond. This bond forges a spirit of cooperation between nursing education and practice, and the benefits are shared in all nursing aspects. Because the preceptor, student, and faculty member, all of whom are integral players in the preceptorship experience, originate from disparate workplace cultures and come together with different resources, they must foster a mutual respect and value what each other can contribute. In doing so, they establish an authentic connection. Open and transparent communication is key to such a union. Regular interactions, explicit sharing of ideas, clarity of expectations, and a focus on areas of strength, as well as those areas requiring improvement, reflect this transparency. Expectations, in particular, must be congruent, so participants from both the practice and the educational settings have a clear understanding of their respective responsibilities/obligations (Puetz &

Shinn, 2002). These expectations must be discussed, agreed on, and written. Specifically, "agreement on financial arrangements, dispute resolution, and communication patterns is a significant component of this step" and is key to laying a strong foundation for a successful partnership (Puetz & Shinn, 2002, p. 182).

The transfer of nursing education from the hospital setting to postsecondary institutions has also brought new challenges, the most compelling of which is the loss of the close association between those nurses who were responsible for teaching and those who were practicing in the field. In other words, a chasm developed between nursing education and nursing practice. This chasm results in a dilemma—the participants on each side are often oblivious to each other, despite the fact that they are

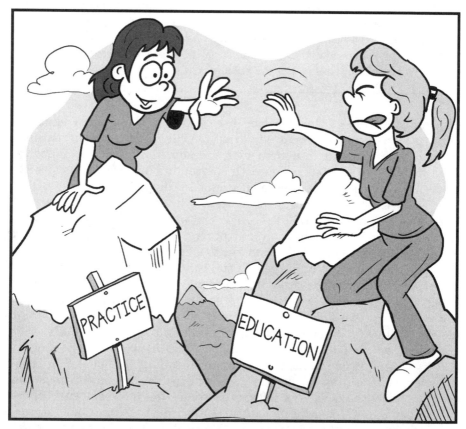

Preceptorship: attempting to bridge the chasm between practice and education.

both ostensibly working toward the shared goal of the provision of the best nursing care possible. However, with the emergence of preceptorship, this chasm can be bridged. Because of the capacity of the preceptorship experience to bridge the gap, it has assumed, albeit fortuitously, a strategic space in the nursing world.

Preceptorship at the Administrative Level

As an approach to clinical teaching, preceptorship pairs a novice with an expert in the practice environment. Such an arrangement affords novice nurses the opportunity to work on a one-to-one basis with expert nurses, who act as resources and who are immediately available to them while they conduct their nursing care. From an administrative perspective, this pairing is the result of a resolute desire on the part of those in nursing education and nursing practice to forge strategic alliances or partnerships that will strengthen the nursing profession. It is at this macro level, between deans/directors and hospital administrators, that formal agreements are negotiated, finalized, and ratified. These formal agreements originally set the stage for the creation of opportunities that help to establish preceptorship as a legitimate teaching-learning experience. Although the basis for such unions are set between the practicing nurse and the individual faculty members and it is within this context that they eventually come to fruition, participants at the administrative level who must support and formalize these partnerships are crucial to the success of the experience. Thus, the importance of the connection between chief nursing officers, deans/directors, department heads, nurse unit managers, etc. cannot be minimized. Those who are directly involved in preceptorship are often completely unaware of the pivotal role that administrators play in the promotion, support, and success of preceptorship as an educational/practice opportunity.

How administrators and managers support preceptors in their teaching role is an integral ingredient of the success of the preceptorship experience. A nurse's primary responsibility is patient care; however, a preceptor also plays a pivotal role in the teaching-learning process. Balancing the two responsibilities can be challenging. Recent research has indicated that preceptors frequently carry unrealistically heavy workloads, which can often leave them little time for teaching (Edmond, 2001). Frequently, preceptors assume charge nurse status, while at the same time assuming their preceptor roles. This predicament can be taxing to the preceptor and preceptee, and to their patients. Being a preceptor is a complex and time-consuming responsibility. It requires educational preparation and support, especially peer support (Kaviani & Stillwell, 2000). Clinical teaching requires considerable teaching skill, and it "cannot be assumed that, by virtue of their knowledge and expertise, practitioners can automatically function as preceptors" (Kaviani & Stillwell, 2000, p. 221). The need for preceptor preparation and support is critical (Yonge, Myrick, Ferguson, & Haase, 2003). Yet, preparation of preceptors is often overlooked or neglected. Adding to this lack of preparation, preceptors are often selected on the basis of their availability and not necessarily on their particular ability for the role (Myrick & Barrett, 1992). Typically, preceptor selection occurs by random assignment. An administrator tells a preceptor "it is your turn" by placing a letter in the potential preceptor's mailbox, asking for volunteers at a staff meeting, posting a notice requesting staff to volunteer, and/or meeting with individual staff and discussing the possibility of being a preceptor. Luckily, some nurses volunteer for the preceptor role and inform the administrator that they want to be considered for that position. The selection process also depends on the depth and involvement of the preceptorship program and can vary in length from a few days to several months.

Regardless of how a nurse becomes a preceptor, organizations and facilities must prepare and accommodate the needs of the nurses who are willing to assume this multidimensional role. Within the landscape of the nursing profession, preceptorship allows for a coalescing of philosophies, ideas, and goals toward the ultimate well-being and good of the profession. In establishing the preceptorship model within a particular organization, administrators must identify their common ground, come to an understanding as to the extent of their organization's commitment, and decide how best to support those directly involved in the preceptorship endeavor. Their sense of commitment to the preparation of future nurses allows them to form a strategic alliance and to establish a climate within which preceptorship can flourish. Preceptorship is a singular dimension of that alliance through which they jointly achieve mutual goals and objectives related to both nursing education and practice. Under the guise of preceptorship, nursing education and nursing practice merge "their respective strengths to achieve compatible objectives while they retain their individual identities and share in risks and rewards" (Puetz & Shinn, 2002, p. 182). The ultimate beneficiary is not only the student, who benefits from the preceptorship experience, but also the preceptor, staff, faculty, and nursing profession in general, who thrive in this combined initiative. Through this approach to clinical or field teaching, the profession prepares its future guardians and leaders. For that reason alone, preceptorship can be considered a pivotal trajectory in the survival of the nursing profession, reflecting even more strongly the role that administrative personnel must assume in making it a priority.

Collaboration Between Faculty and Preceptors

Although the participants at the administrative level lay the formal groundwork for preceptorship, it is between the individual faculty member and the nurse preceptor that the preceptorship experience plays out on a day-to-day, minute-by-minute basis. The intricacies of preceptorship take shape at this juncture. Any form of disconnection at this level can result in considerable consequences for faculty, preceptor, and preceptee. In a recent research study, evidence emerged to indicate that the relationship between the preceptor and the faculty is an important determinant in the development, implementation, and sustainability of the preceptorship experience (Myrick, 1998). In this study, two out of six preceptors expressed dissatisfaction with the relationship, or lack thereof, between themselves and the faculty member with whom they were assigned to work. Their dissatisfaction emanated primarily from a lack of connection with the individual faculty members. The preceptors had expressed concern that the faculty were rarely, if ever, physically present in the practice setting and rarely contacted the preceptors or students throughout the course of the preceptorship experience, which, in this case, was 14 weeks in its entirety. In one particular instance, the preceptor indicated that she finally had to specifically request the learning/course objectives from the preceptee after waiting 3 weeks for the faculty member to provide them. At no time did the faculty member and the preceptor discuss the program, learning objectives, or preceptor and student expectations. Participants must strive to ensure that this type of predicament is avoided if the preceptorship approach to clinical teaching is to continue to survive, much less to thrive, within the context of nursing education and practice.

Faculty Involvement

We cannot ignore how the faculty role has evolved or, more appropriately, devolved, in preceptorship. Although the faculty are not directly involved in teaching preceptored students—and should not be expected to within this approach—they are nevertheless custodians of the teaching-learning process and, therefore, must assume an active role. In other words, their role cannot remain on the periphery of the preceptorship experience, much as it has during the past decade (Myrick, 2002; Yonge, Myrick, Ferguson, & Haase, 2003). Preceptors require that faculty support them by making themselves available, accessible, and willing to be open and authentic in their communication (Gibson & Hauri, 2000). Faculty who are authentic demonstrate a willingness to openly and specifically discuss their expectations of preceptorship as a teaching-learning experience and clarify concerns or questions that may arise and are readily available as a resource to the preceptor. Preceptors need guidance in the teaching-learning process, and faculty members are in the prime position to provide this guidance.

The nurturing of an unfailing commitment by faculty, reflected in their ongoing communication with preceptors and students, is essential to the teaching-learning process. This commitment implies that the faculty are regularly available and accessible throughout the experience. Although it is not always feasible for faculty members to be physically present in the clinical/practice setting, it is essential that the preceptor or student be able to reach them by telephone, pager, or e-mail. Unlike the preceptor who is usually assigned to one or, sometimes, two students, faculty members are often responsible for many students, depending on their particular class size. This high faculty-to-student ratio is often the reason for the faculty member's limited contact. If the connection between the faculty and the preceptor is authentic, the faculty member can communicate this obstacle to the preceptor, and, together, they can make necessary accommodations. However, the communication is crucial. This particular type of connection or collaboration presupposes a certain measure of good will on the part of the involved individuals. The faculty member and preceptor must make a genuine effort not only to connect but also to stay connected, which is sometimes easier said than done. The onus is particularly significant for faculty members. Because of their role as custodians of the teaching/learning process and because they are ultimately responsible for the final evaluation of students involved in the preceptorship experience, faculty members must be diligent and consistent in their efforts to connect with the preceptors and preceptees. Box 1-2 offers a summary of suggestions that faculty can use to promote the connections between faculty and preceptors.

Because the presence of faculty is so important to the successful implementation of the preceptorship experience, it is highly recommended that the faculty establish a regular visitation and communication pattern with units on which the assigned students are being pre-

· ·

Box 1-2

Practical Information: Establishing and Maintaining a Connection—Suggestions for Faculty Members

The faculty member and preceptor must make a genuine effort to not only connect but also stay connected, which is sometimes easier said than done. The following are ways for faculty members to foster a connection.

Establishing a Connection

- Write an orientation and welcome letter to the preceptor that includes information about the preceptorship experience, suggestions concerning the precepting process, and details concerning how best to contact the faculty member.
- Encourage the preceptee to write a letter of introduction to the preceptor and, if possible, send a professional picture.

Meeting With the Preceptor

- Make the effort to meet with the preceptor before the start of the preceptorship experience (if the preceptor is located within commuting distance) and provide the preceptor with both the orientation materials and the student's learning objectives.
- Arrange subsequent meetings as needed.
- Meet at the completion of the preceptorship experience. Include the preceptor, preceptee, and faculty, and focus on the evaluation of the experience.
- For those preceptors who are not within commuting distance (usually more than an hour) telephone calls, faxes, and e-mails are sufficient and essential. Occasionally, other nurse educators living in the area may also volunteer their time and visit the student and preceptor.

Maintaining Communication

- Keep open the lines of communication. Preceptors and students need regular interaction, which can be accomplished through meetings, e-mails, and telephone calls. For any personal contacts, faculty must assess the best times to connect with the preceptor and student.
- Respond to questions from the preceptee or preceptor as soon as possible.
- Acknowledge the preceptor's contribution. At the completion of the rotation, the faculty member should send a detailed letter of acknowledgment to the preceptor with a copy to the student and administrator.

ceptored. Such visits can be used as an opportunity to strengthen the preceptor-faculty relationship, contribute to the teaching-learning process, alleviate any student anxiety, act as support for the preceptee, and facilitate the adjustment period for both the preceptor and the preceptee (Ferguson, 1996; Yonge, Myrick, Ferguson, & Haase, 2003). By making the effort to visit the unit on which the preceptorship experience is occurring, faculty members convey a powerful message to the preceptors, students, and staff. Their action illustrates, even if subliminally, their genuine respect for the contributions made by the preceptors and staff to the preceptees' learning. Their action also implies that the experience is such an important and valued priority that it warrants the personal attention of the faculty. In other words, it is a perceptible or concrete demonstration of the faculty member's commitment to the preceptorship experience and relays the message that preceptorship, as a teaching-learning model, is significant within the academic world.

Although the purpose of the preceptorship experience is to provide an opportunity for preceptees to adapt to the realities of the practice environment, an integral component of that experience is the successful achievement of their learning/program objectives. Therefore, the faculty must ensure that the preceptorship environment is one in which the preceptees' learning can be nurtured appropriately and constructively. Although the preceptor assumes the primary role in teaching the preceptees and introducing them to the ways of nursing practice, remember that the preceptor's priority is patient care. However, the education of preceptees is the priority of the faculty. In a research study on preceptorship (Myrick, 1998), preceptors were "those nurses who so generously give of their time and expertise" (p. 50). The researcher went on to observe:

> It was impressive to witness firsthand how these nurses [preceptors] juggle their preceptor role with their role of staff nurse and/or charge nurse, while at the same time accommodating the learning needs of the nursing students who require much of their time and attention. On more than one occasion, the researcher found herself thinking that these nurses are the "unsung heroes" of the nursing profession, for despite their heavy workloads and complex pressures, they still continue to remain committed to sharing their time, expertise, and the wisdom of their experience with these neophyte nurses. More significantly, they do so in a spirit of true magnanimity (Myrick, 1998, p. 51).

Faculty members must be mindful and recognize the generosity of the preceptors, as well as the major contribution that they continuously make to the educational process. Therefore, faculty members must ensure that they continue to demonstrate their appreciation and, through their actions, remain steadfastly connected and committed to the preceptorship experience. The old adage "actions speak louder than words" is appropriate in this instance.

The connection between faculty and preceptors cannot be overemphasized, because the strength of that relationship directly affects the preceptee. Often, the relationship between the faculty member and preceptor is the first to erode within the preceptorship experience. Therefore, faculty members must be vigilant in establishing this connection and the preceptors must participate in the nurturing of this relationship. Often, the notion that academics live in ivory towers and are out of touch with the real world of nursing prevails. Perpetuation of this myth not only contributes to the erosion of the relationship between faculty and preceptors but also widens the chasm between education and practice. Subsequently, faculty members must make every effort to play a real and visible part in the preceptorship experience.

Preceptor Participation

Although the primary responsibility of the preceptor remains the teaching-learning needs of the preceptee in the practice setting, it is also important that the preceptor maintain regular contact with the faculty. As discussed, communication between the faculty and the preceptor is a pivotal force in the overall success of the preceptorship experience. Although it is important that the faculty assume responsibility in maintaining open communication, it is equally important that the preceptor do likewise. Ideally, the preceptor can begin by meeting with the faculty member and the preceptee immediately before commencement of the preceptorship experience. A face-to-face meeting is preferable. At regular intervals throughout the experience, it is appropriate for the preceptor to connect with the faculty member either directly, if possible, or by telephone or e-mail to discuss the progress of the preceptee and the status of his or her learning objectives. At this time, the faculty member and the preceptor may also address questions and review teaching and learning strategies.

In addition to communicating with the faculty, the preceptor can also encourage the preceptee to connect with the faculty member regularly to discuss his or her progress and to address any concerns regarding the teaching-learning process. By keeping the lines of communication open, the preceptor also can avoid any misunderstandings and deal directly, efficiently, and constructively with any ongoing concerns or questions. Box 1-3 highlights specific actions that the preceptor may take to maintain an authentic connection with the faculty member.

There are multiple dimensions to the world of nursing, including the arenas of clinical practice, research, administration, and education/academia, all of which, although different, comprise the composite referred to as the nursing profession. Each dimension by itself is a necessary but insufficient dimension of the profession. However, together they form a necessary and sufficient whole. By working together, each strengthens

Box 1-3

Practical Information: Connecting—Suggestions for the Preceptor

Although the main focus of the preceptor is orientating the preceptee to the practice setting, the preceptor also must facilitate a connection with the faculty member. The following suggestions help the preceptor to connect.

Establishing a Connection

- Review the information about the preceptee before the commencement of the preceptorship experience. The preceptor should be provided with detailed information about the preceptee, including name, background, learning/program objectives, and a summary of the competencies he or she brings to the experience.
- Discuss who will be supporting you and what form that support will take. If the support derives from a faculty member, aside from the regular/ongoing contact, you must know how to contact that individual faculty member in the event of an emergency.

Keeping Connected

- Ask questions regarding expectations throughout the preceptorship experience.
- Keep the faculty member "in the know." Communicate the status of the preceptee and the experience. Alert him or her to possible problems.
- Enjoy the preceptorship experience, and view it as part of your professional development.

part of the whole, a strengthening that begins with individual relationships that must be nurtured if they are to survive. The same can be said for the preceptorship relationship. By working together collaboratively, the faculty and preceptor can ensure the sustainability of the preceptorship experience and, in turn, contribute to a further solidifying of the nursing profession itself.

• Summary

From both a practice and an academic perspective, shaping the preceptorship experience is challenging. Numerous challenges confront the faculty, preceptors, and preceptees. A successful preceptorship requires a genuine connection of nursing education and practice. To establish and maintain this connection, participants at all levels must commit themselves to the experience. This connection and sharing of resources helps to strengthen both the quality of future nurses and the profession as a whole.

R E F E R E N C E S

Backenstose, A. G. (1983). The use of clinical preceptors. In S. Stuart-Siddall & J. M. Haberlin (Eds.), *Preceptorships in nursing education* (pp. 9–23). Rockville, MD: Aspen Publications.

Chickerella, B. G., & Lutz, W. J. (1981). Professional nurturance: Preceptorship for undergraduate nursing. *American Journal of Nursing, 81*(1), 107–109.

Edmond, C. B. (2001). A new paradigm for practice education. *Nurse Education Today, 21,* 251–259.

Ferguson, L. M. (1996). Preceptors' needs for faculty support. *Journal of Nursing Staff Development, 12*(2), 73–80.

Fernald, D. H., Staudenmaier, A. C., Tressler, C. J., Main, D. S., O'Brien-Gonzales, A., & Barley, G. E. (2001). Students' perspectives on primary care preceptorships: Enhancing the medical student preceptorship learning environment. *Teaching and Learning in Medicine, 13*(1), 13–20.

Gibson, S. E., & Hauri, C. (2000). The pleasure of your company: Attitudes and opinions of preceptors toward nurse practitioner preceptees. *Journal of the American Academy of Nurse Practitioners, 12*(9), 360–363.

Hardyman, R., & Hickey, G. (2001). What do newly qualified nurses expect from preceptorship? Exploring the perspective of the preceptee. *Nurse Education Today, 21,* 58–64.

Kaviani, N., & Stillwell, Y. (2000). An evaluative study of clinical preceptorship. *Nurse Education Today, 20,* 218–226.

Kramer, M. (1974). *Reality shock: Why nurses leave nursing.* St. Louis, MO: C. V. Mosby.

Myrick, F., & Awrey, J. (1988). The effect of preceptorship on the clinical competency of baccalaureate student nurses: A pilot study. *The Canadian Journal of Nursing Research, 20*(3), 29–43.

Myrick, F., & Barrett, C. (1992). Preceptors selection criteria in Canadian basic baccalaureate schools of nursing—A survey. *The Canadian Journal of Nursing Research, 24*(3), 53–64.

Myrick, F. (1998). Preceptorship and critical thinking in nursing education. Unpublished doctoral dissertation. University of Alberta, Edmonton, Alberta.

Myrick, F. (2002). Preceptorship and critical thinking in nursing education. *Journal of Nursing Education, 41*(4), 1154–1164.

Myrick, F., & Yonge, O. (2003). Preceptorship: A quintessential component of nursing education (pp. 91–107). In M. H. Oermann & K. T. Heinrich (Eds.), *Annual Review of Nursing Education* (Vol. 1). New York: Springer.

Puetz, B. E., & Shinn, L. J. (2002). Strategic partnerships. *Journal of Nursing Administration, 32*(4), 182–183.

Usher, K., Nolan, C., Reser, P., Owens, J., & Tollefson, J. (1999). An exploration of the preceptor roles: Preceptors' perceptions of benefits, rewards, supports and commitment to the preceptor role. *Journal of Advanced Nursing, 29*(2), 506–514.

Yonge, O., Myrick, F., Ferguson, L., & Haase, M. (2003). Faculty preparation for the preceptorship experience: The forgotten link. *Nurse Educator 28(5),* 1–2.

CHAPTER 2

The Teaching and Learning Climate

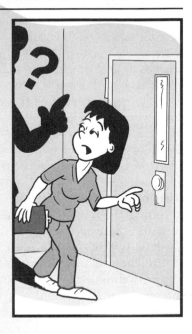

Invariably, many determinants influence the teaching-learning process. One such determinant that is not discussed often but that is always prevalent is the climate, atmosphere, or environment. In this chapter, the term *climate* as it pertains to teaching and learning is discussed. Just as a teacher in a classroom or laboratory setting establishes a climate that is conducive to teaching-learning, a preceptor creates such a climate within the context of the practice setting. However, this climate is not created in isolation from other agency facets. Each person in the agency and every physical structure are parts of the climate. Personnel walking into an agency are immediately aware of the climate, just as a person walking outside is aware of the weather. Comments such as "everyone is busy today" or "things seem a bit hectic" are summaries of impressions, visual cues, and the essence of the workplace.

Even though there is a close relationship between optimal working conditions for personnel and the possibilities for providing good care (Lövgren, Rasmussen, & Engstrom, 2002), little has been written about the climate involving the preceptorship experience. However, in two recent studies in which the fostering of critical thinking between students and preceptors was examined, the climate specifically emerges as being integral to the promotion of student critical thinking (Myrick, 2002; Myrick & Yonge, 2001). For example, one of the studies has found that without a climate of honesty, openness, and security, critical thinking was not possible (Myrick, 2002). The study found that many issues affect the climate, but there are two variables that are central. These variables include the preceptor as the key factor to a constructive climate and the staff who are also an important influence in the process. The preceptors play a pivotal role in influencing the nature of the practice setting and the degree to which the preceptees feel supported in their learning and whether they are subsequently enabled to think critically. The preceptors are instrumental in setting the tone for the learning climate through their attitudes and their ability to work with the preceptees, as opposed to telling them what to do and how to do it. The staff in the practice setting and their acceptance of the preceptees as part of the team affect the climate. In other words, even though the preceptor is the major influence in the climate, others in the setting also have a profound effect on the learning climate (Myrick, 2002). In a second grounded theory study focusing on the enhancement of graduate student critical thinking in the preceptorship experience, a major theme that has emerged as being conductive to a good teaching-learning climate is safety-trust (Myrick & Yonge, in press). Students strongly believe that critical thinking is facilitated only if they have a sense of security when expressing themselves or when questioning the preceptor. Pivotal to that sense of security is both the preceptors' ability to be open to different ways of thinking and their appreciation for the preceptees' opinions. To learn more about clinical education literature and the climate of preceptorship, please see Box 2-1.

• The Ideal Teaching-Learning Climate

Although the learning climate is required to be provocative, stimulating, and disciplined, it should also be a "humanistic one which is authentic, supportive, and caring" (Reilly & Oermann, 1992, p. 45). Sensitivity and caring about the individual preceptee does not automatically preclude an acceptable level of performance or dismiss the notion of clinical competence, but it does imply that the preceptor demonstrates an ongoing commitment to helping preceptees achieve their desired goals and objectives in the practice setting. It also implies that the preceptees' perspectives are encouraged and supported (Myrick & Yonge, 2001).

Box 2-1. Clinical Education Literature

A body of literature regarding clinical education contributes to preceptorship and supports the work of Myrick (2002) and Myrick & Yonge
(2001). Specifically, the most significant factor in establishing a climate
conducive to teaching-learning is the formation of the relationship
between the clinical teacher and student (Nahas, Nour, & Al-Nobani,
1999; Saariskoski, Leino-Kilpi, & Warne, 2002; Woo-Sook, Cholowski, &
Williams, 2002). The accessibility of clinical teachers, their supportive-
ness, and their sensitivity to students' needs contribute to the climate
(Saariskoski et al., 2002). The formation of the relationship is based on
confidence and respect, allowing for freedom of discussion and sharing
of feelings. A clinical teacher who encourages student learning and helps
when needed allows students to be at ease and confident with teachers,
as well as with their new environment (Nahas et al., 1999). Woo-Sook et
al. (2002) discuss two previous studies that report that good interpersonal relationships may be more valuable in the clinical setting than professional competence. Because the learning setting involves such a high
level of stress and uncertainty, a trusting relationship between the clinical
teacher and student is crucial for success (Woo-Sook et al., 2002).
Other factors pertaining to the contributions that teachers or, in this
case, preceptors make to a conducive climate include the use of motiva-
tional principles; critical-thinking strategies; teacher quality management,
including collaboration for the allowance of student control over his or
her learning; clarity of the clinical teacher role; assessment; and an effi-
cient level of competency and knowledge (Massarweh, 1999). The overall
unit or agency climate is also highly significant. Saariskowski et al. (2002)
describe a good unit atmosphere as one that provides individual supervision from a clinical teacher and regular contact between the clinical
teacher and student. Addis and Karadag (2003) state that an effective
ward atmosphere is based on perceiving students as team members.
They further indicate that teaching team membership involves devotion
to individual work with students and regular case discussions that enable
additional knowledge application. Morrow's early work (1984) suggested
that open, nonauthoritarian atmospheres stimulate learner involvement,
initiative, and creativity, which encourage self-confidence and independence.

Perhaps the most renowned teacher and researcher who understood
the adult learner was Malcom Knowles. In nursing education, many

Box 2-1. Clinical Education Literature (*Continued*)

principles regarding teaching and learning have been adapted from his work. In a book that was completed posthumously, Knowles, Holton III, and Swanson (1998) summarized the construction of an effective educative environment. According to these authors, such an environment or climate is based on four particular characteristics: respect for personality/participation in decision making; freedom of expression; availability of information; and mutuality of responsibility in defining goals/planning and conducting activities and evaluating (p. 108). In other words, an educative environment is one that represents democratic values and one in which a democratic philosophy is at play.

• Creating a Hospitable Climate

Just as faculty and preceptors are pivotal to the success of the preceptorship experience, the environment as a whole or the climate in which the experience is played out is also a key factor. "The creation of a positive learning climate has always been a challenge for nurse educators and subsequently has been passed on to preceptors" (Myrick & Yonge, 2001, p. 461). Although the preceptor plays the major role in creating a positive climate in which preceptees can learn and work, the larger environment also significantly affects their experience. Whether the teaching-learning role of the preceptorship experience is genuinely embraced depends, to a large extent, on the philosophic perspective that prevails throughout the setting itself. For example, is the setting one in which education or lifelong learning is valued within the context of clinical/community practice? How open is the setting to student learning? Do staff members in the setting value the contribution that preceptees make to nursing care or do they perceive them to be an additional burden to an already hectic workplace? In other words, is the environment in which the preceptorship experience occurs receptive to the notion of teaching-learning? Is it a welcoming environment? As nurses and educators, we have, at one time or another, assumed the roles of both preceptor and preceptee. Therefore, we can attest to the fact that preceptees frequently find themselves experiencing trepidation when approaching clinical practice and often describe it as being quite daunting. In a recent study, one student described her experience as follows: "You spend so much time walking around on eggshells that you're not thinking up to your capacity" (Myrick, 2002, p. 61). Another preceptee stated, "The happier I am, the more I want to learn" (p. 62). Moreover, the tone that permeates the setting in particular and the organization as a whole can determine how well preceptees surmount the challenges that confront them daily. Ultimately, it is the prevailing attitude of administrators and staff that filters through the organization that contributes to either the alleviation or the enhancement of the trepidation that many preceptees initially experience.

"Hospitality...means primarily the creation of a free space where the stranger can enter and become a friend instead of an enemy. Hospitality is not to change people, but to offer them space where change can take place" (Nouwen, 1975, p. 71). Preceptees must be regarded well by those with whom they interact. They also must know that in their own way they are making a contribution, even if it is small. A recent study (Myrick, 2002) found that preceptees must feel respected, valued, and supported by their preceptors. However, their need to feel accepted by the staff is also important. It is this kind of nurturing atmosphere that fosters a positive learning environment—a climate in which preceptees can thrive. Frequently, preceptees are regarded as guests in the clinical practice setting (Myrick, 1991). Metaphorically, the term *guest* can refer to those who "honor the house with their visit and will not leave it without having made their own contribution" (Nouwen, 1975, p. 89), an interpretation befitting of the involvement of preceptees in the preceptorship experience.

• Factors That Influence the Teaching-Learning Climate

Invariably, there are several factors that influence the teaching-learning environment within the context of the preceptorship experience (Myrick & Yonge, 2001). As we have seen, as the preceptor, you have the greatest impact. You may be perceived as one who is there to "bridge the gap between the reality of the workplace and the idealism of an academic environment without compromising professional ideas" (O'Mara, 1997, p. 57). The preceptees perceive you as their "safety net" or the one person to whom they can turn in times of need. As well, we have also seen that the staff is critical to the success of the preceptee's learning experience. Unless the staff is accepting and supportive of the preceptees, the experience can become quite a challenge for both them and you as their assigned preceptors (Myrick, 2002). All too often the staff can be overlooked as a key to fostering a suitable learning environment. You must always remember the invaluable resource that they contribute to the teaching-learning process. For example, oftentimes when you are busy, it is the staff members who take the preceptees under their wings to help them with their various patient assignments.

Through the years, much has been documented about the significance of the climate as it affects student learning both positively and negatively (Brookfield, 1986; Friere, 1997; Mezirow, 1990). However, most educational experts concur that the climate that is most effective in promoting and enhancing student learning is the environment in which the student is supported and is not made to feel threatened. The climate that is conducive to teaching-learning is one that ultimately reflects an openness that encourages trust and a true spirit of inquiry (Manley, 1997).

The Overall Climate of the Organization

Workload and support strongly affect the energy and the time that you are able to give to a preceptee. If you are swamped with work, understaffed, or required to assume the role of unit charge nurse, it can be quite a challenge to assume the responsibility of preceptor. Preceptees take a considerable amount of time, particularly quality time. Moreover, because of the nature of nurses' work in dealing with vulnerable individuals whose lives may depend on them, it is not advisable or acceptable to provide only superficial supervision. If a preceptee is to be appropriately socialized into the professional role of the nurse, then he or she must be guided in a thoughtfully and vigilantly way. Nursing care is about safety. That safety is guaranteed only through considerable guidance.

Unfortunately, there are times that the people in administration who are there to support you also contribute to your stress (Yonge, Myrick, & Haase, 2002). For example, you might be given a double assignment because you have a student and must assume the role of charge nurse. This situation serves to increase your stress because of the mistaken assumption that your preceptee is a fully functioning professional. When preceptees work under your supervision, they may appear as if they are competent, but this may not always be the case. In fact, preceptees often believe that they have to appear to be confident if they are to succeed in the practice environment. Therefore, it is critical that you make an ardent effort to truly get to know your preceptees. Investing such time will result in your preceptees developing trust in you that, in turn, will allow them to be honest and open about what they can and cannot do. In other words, if you are open with them, then they will not be threatened by you or believe that you will judge them poorly when they need your assistance. Preceptees also resent the loss of preceptors to other duties, especially at the beginning of their rotations. For example, if you are assigned to a preceptee while simultaneously having to assume the charge nurse role, you may be unable to give the preceptee your undivided attention that is so often required in the teaching-learning process. Preceptees who are faced with such a situation often feel disadvantaged. They also believe that they may be a bother to you in the middle of your "more important" nursing responsibilities. Another situation that could complicate the assignment of preceptors is the preceptee who is employed in the agency in another capacity or role, for example, the student who works on the unit on weekends and holidays as a nursing assistant and who, therefore, is not perceived in the student role or regarded by others as being a student. Staff members may have difficulty discerning when the student is in the preceptee role or in the nursing assistant role. Under such circumstances, it is not unusual for students to feel resentful if they are being used as an employee when they need and want to be learners. The preceptees may understand their role, but the person who is responsible for patient assignments could be more concerned with obtaining adequate staffing and, therefore, neglect to consider their learning needs as preceptees. Instead, they are given responsibilities that make no contribution to their learning.

Emotional Climate

Another issue that may affect the climate is the emotional exhaustion of the staff (Stordeur, D'Hoore, & Vandenberghe, 2001). When agencies are experiencing difficulty in recruiting or retaining staff, the end result can be increased stress for the remaining staff. Other obstacles, such as working under constraints with a reduced number of staff, extensive structural change, or a discrepancy between work demands and resources, may also affect the climate (Lövgren et al., 2002). Using the Nursing Stress Scale, Stordeur et al. found that 22% of the variance for 625 nurses resulted from emotional exhaustion. This factor had the greatest variance. Nurses reported that they found their physical and social environments, unclear roles, and particular leadership styles to be highly stressful. If you believe that you are emotionally exhausted and have a choice whether to accept a preceptee, it is important that you reflect first on your own needs.

Agencies often inform nurses/teachers about a preceptorship program through e-mail or written communication, but others use a more consultative style by inquiring as to who would like to be a preceptor.

Some administrators believe that staff members should alternate the role of preceptor while actually communicating indirectly that being assigned to a preceptee can be stressful and burdensome. Even though alternating the preceptor role between nurses might be preferable, there are instances in which it would be helpful for a preceptor to be assigned to two consecutive preceptees, particularly if the preceptor wishes to develop specific teaching skills. Therefore, it is important that you, as the preceptor, decide if you are ready and able emotionally to teach a preceptee. Your emotions set the stage for the learning climate. You are the major vehicle or means for teaching in the preceptorship experience, and if you are feeling emotionally exhausted, you will either directly or indirectly communicate this to the preceptee.

Another aspect of the creation of the teaching-learning climate involves the one constructed by the preceptee. In reviewing the literature regarding undergraduate student stress and the clinical environment, Elliot (2002) found that student nurse stress is greater than the stress of students in allied health professions (DiGiacomo & Adamson, 2001). Interestingly, students described several fears: harming the patient, feeling inadequate because of inexperience and lack of knowledge, general feelings of incompetence, failing, and unknown. Because they are learners, preceptees fear making mistakes. As students, they possess a limited knowledge base and, consequently, doubt their own ability to work safely and confidently. They also fear you, the preceptor. They ask themselves: What will you be like? Will you want them as your student? Will you be fair, tolerant, and helpful? Will they get along with you? They bring with them a host of potential negative emotions that could adversely affect the climate. Some preceptees may appear overly confident or even boastful, but really they may be attempting to hide their fears and, because of their behavior, may only irritate those around them. For example, some preceptees who are particularly fearful or anxious may talk too much or respond inappropriately in a serious situation. For example, have you ever worked with a preceptee who laughed in a particularly sad or solemn situation? Such inappropriate behavior may be an indication of just how fearful or inadequate they may really feel.

Because preceptees are always a presence with you as you work throughout your shifts, you may feel that you have acquired another physical shadow. This can be problematic at the beginning of the placement, because preceptees require a considerable amount of direction and attention. Also, when preceptees cannot be trusted, are not motivated, or have extremely limited clinical skills, you may also find yourself particularly taxed (Yonge, Krahn, Trojan, Reid, & Haase, 2002). You might even begin to feel resentful toward the preceptee or feel used by others. If you

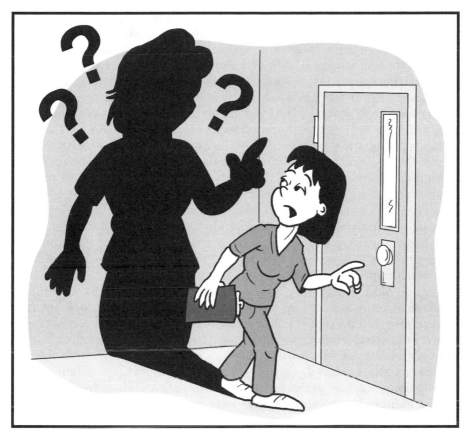

At times, the preceptee may feel like a shadow, constantly following you around.

experience these feelings, it is extremely important that you seek support from those in management or administrative positions. If the preceptee is a student, his or her educational institution contact personnel must be notified. Do not, for 1 minute, believe that you are isolated and that the burden of precepting is your sole responsibility.

Physical Environment

As nurses, we accept the physical working environment. We treat the environment as a given. It may be noisy, bright, dull, crowded, and so forth, and we accept the environment for what it is and work in and around it. According to Lövgren et al. (2002), the work climate not only affects the comfort and well-being of the employees but also the potential innovative capacity within the agency. If the agency is an older building, it may not have been designed to accommodate all the needs of the various health care workers, such as occupational health or physiotherapy. The charting room may be small and crowded, even without the addition of a preceptee. If the agency is without walls (eg, home health care or community care agencies) and you use your vehicle to visit patients, you may not have vehicle insurance to cover the cost of a preceptee. This may mean juggling your visitation schedule around available transportation times for the preceptee. There may also be sensitivities about being accompanied by a preceptee on your visits, because he or she may be viewed as a stranger in a community agency. Patients who are admitted into agencies that are designated as "teaching hospitals" tolerate or even welcome interactions with several students. As a home care or community health nurse, particularly in the mental health area, you may have taken months to establish a relationship, and the relationship might be quickly disrupted if a preceptee accompanies you.

Crowding in agencies is also an issue. There may be insufficient space to accommodate all of the different learners or preceptees. You may be assigned to a preceptee and may wish to provide this person with several learning experiences and opportunities, only to discover that there is a designated clinical educator in your agency who is responsible for numerous students. Subsequently, you and your preceptee may not be able to access certain patients. Given the rise of specialties in health care, access to fundamental nursing care opportunities is at a premium.

• Preceptors' Responsibilities for Influencing the Climate

As a preceptor, your first priority is patient care. However, you are also involved in and responsible for teaching a preceptee how to deliver this care. As discussed, one of the most significant factors in establishing a positive teaching-learning climate is the relationship that is formed with the student. This climate is established by first reflecting on the type of relationship in which you would like to engage, your own learning style, your workload, and the support others in the agency are willing to offer you. There are also degrees of intimacy in a relationship that range from warm to cool. Some preceptors prefer to work closely with the preceptee. This approach is referred to as side-by-side learning. Others prefer a hands-off style, where there is a short meeting at the commencement of the shift and again during the check-out at the end of the shift. In this less intimate relationship, the preceptor is available to the preceptee only if there is a problem or question.

Setting the Tone of the Relationship

When initially meeting preceptees, it is usually best to meet with them away from the agency and to allow sufficient time for you to get to know each other. Preceptees bring their own sets of skills and abilities. Ask your preceptees what they want to learn, what is the best method of supervision for them, and what would be the best way to work with them. Be clear about your style of interaction, and ask the preceptee if he or she has a preferred style.

In a preceptorship arrangement, the teacher-student relationship is particularly significant. For example, there may be only one or two preceptees per preceptor, thus the physical closeness of the preceptee is part of the relationship and the relationship is public. Other agency personnel know that you are a preceptor and are frequently curious about the preceptee and how you are working with him or her. If administration is interested in recruiting the preceptee, there may be even more scrutiny.

One fundamental aspect to this relationship is feedback. If the preceptees are students, they are used to and interested in receiving feedback regarding their performance. They require both positive and negative feedback. This is a skill that in your role as a nurse you do not typically use when giving patient care. Consequently, giving excessive, insufficient, or negative feedback can result in conflict between you, as the preceptor, and the student. If you give the preceptee daily feedback in a private location, the preceptee will usually feel more secure. As a preceptor, you must know what type of feedback the preceptee requires. This is best accomplished if the preceptee develops a list of objectives that are revised weekly or biweekly. You and the preceptee require structure for giving and receiving feedback. The reverse also is often true. You will also want feedback from the preceptees about how you are teaching. Preceptees are used to providing feedback to clinical teachers, but they usually only do so on a confidential evaluation form. Students welcome the opportunity to give feedback but must be encouraged to do so.

Maintaining the Relationship

In the preceptor-preceptee relationship, there is an inherent power imbalance. Preceptees need to learn, but they need to do so safely. They also need to take responsibility for their own learning. If you are always saying to a preceptee, "it is time for you to have more patients" or "by lunch you should have accomplished more," then the preceptees may not be taking responsibility. This behavior is to be expected as preceptees orient to the agency. Part of taking responsibility is having opportunities to be responsible. You need to trust that the preceptees will be safe in assuming their assignments and that their actions will produce an effective outcome for themselves and the patients. If it takes a preceptee 2 hours to change a simple dressing, then the patient is compromised.

Another important component of the relationship is collaboration. Most preceptor-preceptee relationships thrive because preceptors know how to work as part of a collaborative and cooperative team. As a preceptor, you know the importance of working together on a team (eg, in instances when procedures call for more than one person, such as the two-person lift or coverage for meals). Preceptees may have the same collaborative skills, such as listening to each other, helping beyond a patient assignment, giving feedback, or covering for each other. They learn these skills as you and others in the agency model these behaviors. Frequently, you may need to teach appropriate behavior. Preceptees may also experience difficulty recognizing that they should be assisting others with work assignments, particularly if they are feeling overwhelmed with their own assignment.

All preceptees want to feel confident, which eventually will enable them to function independently. They know they need your teaching, guidance, support, and coaching to help them, but by the end of the rotation, they want to feel and believe that they have acquired knowledge that renders them capable of providing safe, ethical, and competent patient care (Lofmark & Wikblad, 2001). To accomplish this goal, they also need exposure to several patient care experiences. Although being assigned to the same patient for 3 weeks, for example, may give preceptees continuity, it may also serve to undermine their self-confidence. They may also need experiences with wider work systems, such as giving reports or team leading. Providing new experiences and learning opportunities contributes to a climate of constant learning.

Terminating the Preceptorship Experience Positively

Time is needed to start the relationship and to terminate it. In a climate that is conducive to teaching-learning, it is essential that the preceptorship experience begin, proceed, and end positively and constructively. If you have invested a great deal of time in the preceptee and have formed a strong bond, it will be natural for you to experience a loss when the relationship terminates. Usually the formal evaluation of the preceptee provides a method of officially ending the relationship. Preceptees may offer a gift as a symbol of their appreciation for the extra work that you have done for them and the time that you have committed to their learning. They may also give a gift to all the staff in recognition of the support that they received from the team. Also, it is not uncommon for preceptors to give small gifts to their preceptees in recognition of the pleasure that they derived from the experience of having been a preceptor. Although preceptors acknowledge that they may have been involved in teaching preceptees, they also recognize that they have learned from the preceptees, particularly by responding to their many questions and challenges.

If the relationship has been difficult and the preceptee evaluation is marginal, often a great deal of stress is created for the preceptor. Or, if the evaluation has a significant impact on the preceptees' career progression, they may criticize or even formally appeal the preceptor's written evaluation. Preceptees may blame preceptors for their poor performance, lack of insight into their own skills, attitude, or knowledge, or cite certain circumstances that affected their personal lives, such as a breakup with a boyfriend or girlfriend.

The stress of the preceptorship experience may also cause preceptees to act unacceptably and inappropriately (Yonge et al., 2002). Regardless of the quality of the relationship between the preceptor and preceptee, the experience must end with dignity and critical appraisal. Preceptees must be informed, constructively and appropriately, about what went wrong and why. For example, there are preceptees who should not be allowed to complete a rotation because they are not able to master the skills required of them to give safe nursing care within a reasonable time frame. Occasionally, preceptees are nurtured and given the benefit of the doubt because of their student status, only to discover later that they fail a rotation or are asked to leave an agency. Occasionally, preceptees may assert that because they have a right to learn, a failing or unsatisfactory evaluation is not justified, especially if they have been allowed to complete the rotation. As a preceptor, you must be prepared for such eventualities so that from the beginning and throughout the preceptorship experience you can establish an environment that circumvents such occurrences from happening. As discussed, if you create a climate that fosters respect and trust on the part of the preceptee, it is less likely that such situations will occur.

• Summary

As discussed, the climate or environment in which the preceptorship experience occurs is a critical factor in the teaching-learning process. The key factor in creating a climate that is conducive to that process is the formation or establishment of a professional relationship between the preceptor and preceptee. That relationship involves three stages, which include the initial or beginning, the middle or maintenance process, and the closing or termination of the relationship or experience. Throughout those stages, many variables or factors confound the nature or evolution of the preceptorship experience. Inherent in the climate are key factors, such as yourself as the preceptor, the staff members who contribute to much of the preceptees' experiences, and the overall milieu that exists within the particular unit or agency in which the preceptorship takes place. The preceptees bring preconceived notions and remnants of previous situations to the preceptorship experience that can affect all phases of the process. Because of their inexperience, they also may possess many fears that can often affect their behavior in several ways, which can be detrimental to their relationship with you. In the final phase or stage of the preceptorship experience, the formal evaluation must be gentle and constructive. It is critical that both you and your preceptee walk away from the experience with a sense of achievement.

REFERENCES

Addis, G., & Karadag, A. (2003). An evaluation of nurses' clinical teaching role in Turkey. *Nurse Education Today, 23*, 27–33.

Brookfield, S. D. (1986). *Understanding and facilitating adult learning: A comprehensive analysis of principles and effective practices*. San Francisco: Jossey-Bass.

DiGiacomo, M., & Adamson, B. (2001). Coping with stress in the workplace: Implications for new health professionals. *Journal of Allied Health, 30*, 106–111.

Elliott, M. (2002). The clinical environment: A source of stress for undergraduate nurses. *Australian Journal of Advanced Nursing, 20*, 34–38.

Friere, P. (1997). *Pedagogy of the oppressed* (rev ed.). New York: Continuum.

Knowles, M. S., Holton III, E. H., & Swanson, R. A. (1998). *The adult learner* (5th ed.). Houston, TX: Gulf Publishing Company.

Lofmark, A., & Wikblad, K. (2001). Facilitating and obstructing factors for development of learning in clinical practice: A student perspective. *Journal of Advanced Nursing, 34*(1), 430–450.

Lövgren, G., Rasmussen, B. H., & Engstrom, B. (2002). Working conditions and the possibility of providing good care. *Journal of Nursing Management, 10*, 201–209.

Manley, M. S. (1997). Adult learning concepts important to precepting. In J. B. Flynn (Ed.), *The role of the preceptor: A guide for nurse educators and clinicians* (pp. 15–47). New York: Springer.

Massarweh, L. J. (1999). Promoting a positive clinical experience. *Nurse Educator, 24*(3), 44–47.

Mezirow, J. (1990). *Fostering critical reflection in adulthood: A guide to transformative and emancipatory learning.* San Francisco: Jossey-Bass.

Morrow, K. L. *Preceptorships in nursing staff development.* (1984). Rockville, MD: Aspen.

Myrick, F. (1991). The plight of clinical teaching in baccalaureate nursing education. *Journal of Nursing Education, 30*(1), 44–46.

Myrick, F. (2002). Preceptorship and critical thinking nursing education. *Journal of Nursing Education, 41*(4), 154–154.

Myrick, F., & Yonge, O. (2001). Creating a climate for critical thinking in the preceptorship experience. *Nurse Education Today, 21,* 461–467.

Myrick, F., & Yonge, O. (in press). Enhancing critical thinking in the preceptorship experience. *Journal of Advanced Nursing.*

Nahas, V. L., Nour, V., & Al-Nobani, M. (1999). Jordanian undergraduate nursing students' perceptions of effective clinical teachers. *Nurse Education Today, 19,* 639–648.

Nouwen, H. (1975). *Reaching out: The three movements of the spiritual life.* Garden City, MO: Doubleday.

O'Mara, A. (1997). A model preceptor program for student nurses. In J. P. Flynn (Ed.), *The role of the preceptor. A guide for nurse educators and clinicians* (pp. 47–75). New York: Springer.

Reilly, D. E., & Oermann, M. H. (1992). *Clinical teaching in nursing education* (2nd ed.). New York: National League for Nursing.

Saariskoski, M., Leino-Kilpi, H., & Warne, T. (2002). Clinical learning environment and supervision: Testing a research instrument in an international comparative study. *Nurse Education Today, 22,* 340–349.

Stordeur, S., D'Hoore, W., & Vandenberghe, C. (2001). Leadership, organizational stress, and emotional exhaustion among hospital nursing staff. *Journal of Advanced Nursing, 35*(4), 533–542.

Yonge, O., Krahn, H., Trojan, L., Reid, D., & Haase, M. (2002). Being a preceptor is stressful! *Journal for Nurses in Staff Development, 18*(1), 22–27.

Yonge, O., Myrick, F., & Haase, M. (2002). Student nurse stress in the preceptorship experience. *Nurse Educator, 27*(2), 84–88.

Woo-Sook, C. L., Cholowski, K., & Williams, A. K. (2002). Nursing students' and clinical educators' perceptions of characteristics of effective clinical educators in an Australian university school of nursing. *Journal of Advanced Nursing, 39*(5), 412–420.

CHAPTER 3

The Players

Role and Responsibilities

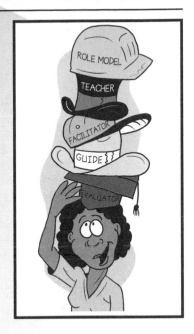

T he preceptorship experience involves three key players—the preceptor, the student/preceptee, and the faculty member. Combined, these players often are referred to as a triad. Each member of this triad plays a critical part in the success of the preceptorship experience. However, the preceptorship relationship is only as strong as its weakest link. Therefore, all three players must work well together to ensure the best possible preceptorship experience. Staff who work in units involved in preceptorship also contribute to the experience. Although they are often considered peripheral to the preceptorship experience, staff members are an integral factor to its success. Preceptorship connects practice and education. For this connection to work, players from both sides must understand their roles. Each player assumes many roles; each role involves several intrinsic responsibilities. For each role in this chapter, a *Practical Information Box* that highlights the responsibilities generally associated with that role is included. (We use the word *generally* because these responsibilities may vary according to different program objectives.)

• The Practice Players

Preceptor

As preceptor, in addition to assuming patient care responsibilities, you must assume a *pivotal* role in the teaching-learning process. Your part in the preceptorship experience requires you to serve as *role model, teacher, facilitator, guide*, and *evaluator* and, in the true sense of the word, assume the *guardianship* of individual preceptees who are often neophytes or novices in the practice arena. Therefore, the preceptor position is multifaceted. For clarity, we explore the many roles that comprise your preceptor responsibility. (See Appendix A for frequently asked questions.)

Role Model

Generally, the term *role model* denotes a particular individual whose style, behavior, way of speaking, and thinking we would inevitably like to emulate or imitate. When the term *role model* is broached with preceptees, they often depict their preceptor as the person with whom they would most like to identify professionally. Preceptees usually want to emulate their preceptors. Traditionally, role modeling has been not only an accepted way to teach professional behaviors and attitudes but also acknowledged as one of the most powerful ways by which learning occurs in the practice setting (Betz, 1985; Bidwell & Brasler, 1989; Davis, 1993; Howie, 1988; Infante, Forbes, Houldin, & Naylor, 1989; Myrick, 1998). In the preceptorship experience, the preceptor serves as a powerful role model for the preceptee. As preceptor, you play the *major* role in the success or failure of the preceptee's experience.

What does it mean to be a role model to a preceptee? Being a role model means that you have a real sense of what it is to be a professional and that you readily translate that sense into your everyday actions in the practice environment. It means that you have a strong commitment to your work and that your manner or demeanor reflects this commitment. As a registered nurse, you serve in a professional capacity while providing nursing care to patients and their families. How you interact with your colleagues, your patients, their families, physicians, and other members of the health care team reflects your sense of professionalism. Preceptees (especially if they are beginners) observe, internalize, and frequently mirror this reflection in their own behaviors.

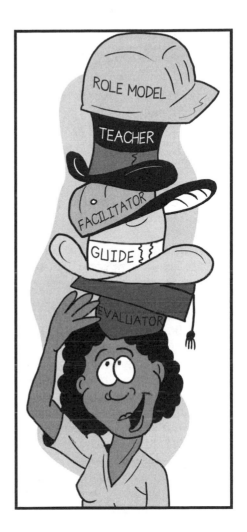

The preceptor wears many hats.

To be an effective role model for preceptees, the preceptor must keep several key criteria in mind. *First*, as mentioned, to be a role model is to be a professional. Your actions, specifically the manner in which you interact with colleagues, patients, families, physicians, and other health care professionals, demonstrate your professionalism. How you interact with others makes a lasting impression on preceptees, especially if they are novices. To be a professional is also to be knowledgeable about the

• • • • • • • • • • • • • • • • • •

B o x   3 - 1

Practical Information: Responsibilities as Role Model

As preceptor, you are responsible for role modeling what it means to be a professional. You fulfill this responsibility by:

- Demonstrating a strong sense of commitment to your role as a nurse and as preceptor
- Interacting with colleagues, patients/clients, families, physicians, and other members of the health care team adeptly and sensitively
- Being knowledgeable about the work that you do
- Exhibiting respect for your patients and coworkers
- Adhering to ethical principles in carrying out your nursing care
- Fostering a spirit of inquiry and critical thinking/reflecting when working with preceptees and colleagues

---

work you do and to be respectful of your patients and your coworkers. To be a professional is to be ethical in your practice, to be prudent or careful in your clinical judgments, and to possess a large measure of practical wisdom. *Second*, your knowledge, expertise, and experience serve as the foundation for your role. Preceptees look to you for your ability to handle situations and put considerable faith in your wisdom as a practitioner. *Third*, your ability to consider clinical situations with an open mind and from several perspectives will enable preceptees to develop their own critical-thinking abilities.

A major part of role modeling involves your ability to think critically while carrying out nursing care. We describe critical thinking as your capacity to consider a patient or clinical situation from several different perspectives and your ability to form a judgment about what to do or what to believe in that particular instance (Facione & Facione, 1996). A recent study that involved fourth-year basic baccalaureate nursing students and their staff nurse preceptors in the acute care setting found that preceptors role model critical thinking directly *and* indirectly through their everyday behaviors (Myrick, 2002). In other words, as you go about your daily nursing care, preceptees find that they are enabled to think critically when (1) they observe the way you deal with the many situations with which you are confronted, (2) you share your ideas with them about how and why you behave and make decisions the way you do in such situations, and (3) you encourage them to voice their own ideas and questions regarding the different occurrences that they encounter.

Teacher

In your position as staff nurse, you constantly interact with patients and their families to convey information concerning patient status and to share your professional perspective regarding issues related to health promotion and illness prevention. As a preceptor, the teacher focus assumes a slightly different direction. Now, instead of sharing knowledge and information only with patients and their families, you will share your knowledge and expertise with your preceptees. However, there is a major stipulation: you will *not* be responsible for teaching program content to preceptees. Such responsibility will remain strictly under the jurisdiction of the faculty member, who will also act as your resource and support person regarding matters pertaining to the teaching-learning process.

The purpose of the preceptorship experience is to provide a one-to-one relationship in which you, as the preceptor, and the preceptee can work closely together in providing nursing care. This one-to-one relationship provides preceptees with a critical sense of security while they are learning in a complex environment that can be daunting. One preceptee described the preceptorship as the "safety net" in the practice setting (Myrick, 2002). When situations become challenging or unmanageable for preceptees, they find comfort knowing that they can turn to you for help and direction. If you are paired with beginning students, you may find that they require constant supervision, facilitation, and guidance when conducting their var-

• • • • • • • • • • • • • • • • • • • •

Box 3-2

Practical Information: Responsibilities as Teacher

Part of preceptorship is sharing knowledge and expertise with your preceptees by

- Supervising preceptees when planning, implementing, and evaluating their nursing care
- Adhering to principles of teaching-learning theories when instructing preceptees
- Using the preceptees' learning and program objectives to guide the teaching-learning process
- Encouraging the preceptees to think critically
- Providing the preceptees with opportunities to try skills and apply their knowledge

ious responsibilities. As they gain more confidence and become increasingly competent, they will, under your expert supervision, develop greater independence and require less of your time and attention.

To maximize your role as teacher, it is particularly important for you to become familiar with various mechanisms designed to help you facilitate the teaching-learning process. These mechanisms provide you with insights into the use of several teaching strategies that will assist you in (1) selecting appropriate patient assignments, (2) promoting the preceptees' ability to think critically, (3) implementing effective and useful evaluation techniques, (4) using principles of teaching and learning, and (5) using student development theory. Such knowledge provides you with the requisite skills needed to become effective in your role as teacher and, hopefully, will result in a more rewarding and successful preceptorship for both you and your preceptees. Please refer to Chapter Five for a detailed discussion.

Facilitator

An equally important component of serving as preceptor is that of facilitation. To *facilitate* means *to make easy* (Concise Oxford Dictionary, 1982). As a facilitator in the preceptorship experience, you draw on your expertise and experience to assist preceptees in achieving their learning goals and objectives (Beckett & Wall, 1985). In the practice setting, preceptees find themselves in a vulnerable position. Consider the following:

Box 3 - 3

Practical Information: Responsibilities as Facilitator

The preceptor must assist preceptee progress throughout the preceptorship experience by:

- Being collaborative and not directive when instructing preceptees
- Using additional resources within the practice setting to benefit the preceptees' experience
- Ensuring that preceptees are appropriately prepared for their patient assignments
- Adopting a positive approach to preceptees
- Encouraging open communication with preceptees

as preceptees in the practice setting, their learning occurs as a public event in front of numerous individuals, including the person for whom they are supposed to be caring, the patient. Preceptees must conduct their learning and develop competency in front of not only you, their preceptor, but also their peers, other patients, various health care workers, agency staff, and often even individuals from other disciplines (Reilly & Oermann, 1992). As a facilitator, you essentially become *a manager of learning.* This requires you to address preceptees' needs, interests, and abilities; to establish a means for formal and informal discussion with preceptees; and to demonstrate ongoing support in what is a frequently threatening and always complex environment.

There are several means at your disposal that will serve to help you facilitate. *First,* use the preceptees' learning and program objectives as a framework with which to organize the preceptorship experience. By providing several experiences that will assist the preceptee in achieving these objectives, you facilitate their learning. *Second,* be mindful of being collaborative and *not* directive in your relationship with your preceptees. Sometimes when you are working with beginning preceptees, it is much easier to tell them how to do something or what and when to do it than to encourage them to think critically. However, such an approach is contrary to the notion of facilitation. Preceptees must believe that you respect and value their perspective, and a collaborative approach on your part provides a sense of working together that can, in turn, not only assist preceptees in their learning but also contribute greatly to their developing confidence and competence. *Third,* use any additional resources that are available to you in the practice setting. Frequently, you can use opportunities that arise to your advantage. For example, if someone on your unit is performing a procedure that would be beneficial to your preceptee's learning, try to have your preceptee participate in it in some way. Have your preceptees attend rounds to provide them with a sense of how the health care team enters into discussion regarding patient status and progress. Many other opportunities can arise within this context. *Fourth,* get into the habit of planning or preparing the preceptee. This can be conducted formally through preconferences and postclinical conferences or informally, but still effectively, through discussions and conversations in the practice environment. *Fifth,* encourage the preceptees. Although they may not often verbalize it, many preceptees, particularly if they are beginning students, are terrified in the practice setting. Preceptees may experience insomnia the night before their clinical practicum and often develop physical symptoms as a result of their increased anxiety. Your encouragement is a key component in alleviating their anxiety and is a major contributory factor to their success in the overall preceptorship experience. *Finally*, remember that you are also there to evaluate the preceptee's performance and are accountable for ensuring that you are accurate and fair in that process. Please refer to the section on the evaluator role for additional discussion.

Guide

When you guide preceptees, you advise them or *show them the way* in their practice experience (Concise Oxford Dictionary, 1982). As a preceptor, you guide preceptees on a daily basis in several ways. *First*, by selecting meaningful learning experiences, you guide preceptees in the teaching-learning process. For example, in considering the appropriateness of patient assignments that the preceptee's learning objectives' require and by ensuring that such assignments are available, you guide preceptees by focusing on specific areas of learning. *Second*, when you provide preceptees with opportunities to develop their psychomotor competencies and advise them in perfecting these skills, you guide their learning. For example, you will often discover that some preceptees are eager to participate in procedures that are new to them, whereas others may be reticent or reluctant to complete a particular procedure because of their lack of confidence. In each instance, it is your responsibility to assess the preceptees' capabilities and to provide guidance as to the appropriate action to be taken, in this case whether to participate, that is in the best interests of the preceptee and, ultimately, the patient. *Third*, as you complete

---

B o x   3 - 4

Practical Information: Responsibilities as Guide

As preceptor, you are responsible for guiding the preceptee throughout various aspects of the preceptorship experience by:

• Providing patient assignments that are appropriate to the level of preceptees' experience and their individual capabilities
• Advising preceptees on the most effective manner in which to improve various competencies
• Showing preceptees how to best develop their problem-solving and clinical decision-making skills
• Opening up opportunities for additional learning experiences

the decision-making and problem-solving processes in patient situations, you help guide preceptees to develop their clinical decision-making and problem-solving skills. *Finally,* when you give preceptees immediate feedback about their performance, you show them how to modify their actions so that it will benefit their own professional development, as well as their patients' well-being (Bizek & Oermann, 1990; Myrick, 2002). As a result of your guidance in each of these areas, you contribute immeasurably to the important process of socializing preceptees into the art of nursing and the realm of professional practice.

Evaluator

Perhaps one of the most challenging aspects of the preceptor role is that of evaluator. To evaluate means to *judge,* and, in this case, you are in the primary position for judging the clinical competence of the preceptees for whom you serve as preceptor. It is important to note that although as a preceptor you may find the evaluation process to be challenging, the preceptees who you evaluate may/will find the process both challenging and threatening. From the preceptees' perspective, the fate of their practice experience rests primarily in your hands. Therefore, it is incumbent on you to be fair, accurate, and, most of all, gentle, throughout this sensitive and vulnerable process.

Resulting from the complexity of nursing practice and the numerous competencies that require preceptee mastery, the evaluator role requires you to use several techniques to assist you with the evaluation

---

B o x   3 - 5

Practical Information: Responsibilities as Evaluator

The preceptor fulfills his or her role as evaluator by:

- Being fair and equitable in conducting your evaluation responsibilities
- Using the preceptees' learning objectives when evaluating student performance
- Consulting with preceptees daily to discuss areas of strength and areas that require improvement
- Ensuring that preceptees have input into their evaluation
- Encouraging self-evaluation

process. These techniques include *direct observation, verbal feedback, written feedback, anecdotal recording, critical incident reports*, and the use of a *rating scale, checklist,* and *self-evaluation.* We explore these techniques in Chapter Eight.

Guardian

Finally, your role in assuming the guardianship of preceptees is significant in the preceptorship experience. Your continuous and consistent support is integral to that role. As a preceptor, you are particularly influential in establishing the degree of support that preceptees receive throughout their learning experience. For example, a practice setting that has abundant learning experiences but lacks support may be extremely discouraging and demoralizing for preceptees and may result in the loss of many opportunities for growth (Myrick, 2002; Myrick & Yonge, 2001; Reilly & Oermann, 1992). You cannot overestimate the effect of your support on preceptees. You must be aware of subtle group dynamics in the practice setting and, subsequently, modify the environment accordingly to allow preceptees to reach an acceptable level of comfort, an essential factor to a successful learning experience. Also, the preceptor is in a key position to raise staff awareness of the dynamics involved and facilitate staff consciousness by presenting a positive model of cordiality, acceptance, and hospitality to preceptees (Myrick & Yonge, 2001).

B o x   3 - 6

Practical Information: Responsibilities as Guardian

As preceptor you act as guardian to the preceptee by:

- Demonstrating support and consistency
- Being aware of the subtle group dynamics on the unit that affect the preceptee's performance
- Making necessary changes, where possible, to create a learning climate that is conducive to the teaching-learning process and optimizing the preceptee's practical experience
- Being cordial, accepting, and hospitable

The Staff

Although the preceptor assumes the primary role in the preceptorship experience, there can be no mistaking the secondary, yet crucial, role that the staff assumes. The preceptor is the major influence on the preceptee experience in the practice setting; staff members in the setting also affect the learning climate and, subsequently, can enhance or impede that experience. Staff members include anyone from the nurse unit manager to the staff nurse, from the physician to the physiotherapist, from the house-keeper to the ward clerk (Myrick, 2002). Staff attitude is particularly significant. Often, a new face on a nursing unit can be cause for alarm and can create a sense of uncertainty for members of the nursing and ancillary staffs. New faces can be indicative of new ideas, which may mean change, that can be threatening to established staff (Myrick & Yonge, 2001). Although preceptee input is meant to be helpful, staff may interpret this as a form of criticism or intrusiveness. Subsequently, the fallout in the defensive nature of the staff can have disastrous results for the well-meaning preceptees. During the preceptorship experience, staff play the learning resource and supporter roles.

Learning Resource

Staff members can serve as major learning resources for preceptees in the preceptorship experience. The staff comprise a large component of the

---

B o x   3 - 7

Practical Information: Responsibilities as Learning Resource

The staff may act as a resource to the preceptee and the staff nurse preceptor by:

- Responding to questions and concerns from both the preceptor and the preceptees
- Facilitating the preceptor's role regarding the selection of appropriate patient assignments
- Offering assistance with patient assignments when required
- Contributing to the overall support of learning experiences

expertise from which preceptees can benefit throughout their learning experience in the practice setting. A primary factor that encroaches on that experience is the relationship between the preceptor and the staff. The preceptor's relationship with his or her colleagues and other members of the health care team often directly affects the preceptees. If the preceptor has a good working relationship with the staff, then such a dynamic can positively affect the preceptee experience. As one student so aptly recounts, "I guess [be]cause the staff respect her it amazingly rubs off on me" (Myrick, 2002, p. 160).

Because of their experience, expertise, and knowledge, the staff possess several helpful skills that provide a key learning resource to the preceptee in the practice setting. Although preceptees essentially work one-on-one with their assigned preceptors, they are nevertheless exposed to and frequently avail themselves of the expertise of several staff members with whom they come into contact in their daily experience. In other words, it is not unusual for different members of the health team to provide a major source of learning. Often, nursing staff accommodates preceptees when new procedures are being conducted on the unit. If a new patient is being admitted to the unit and is under the care of a nurse other than the student's assigned preceptor, it is not uncommon for that nurse to include preceptees in the admission procedure, particularly if they have not yet had such an opportunity. Another example is the case of the physiotherapist who, while providing a regimen of deep breathing exercises with a patient, accommodates the preceptee's learning needs by demonstrating the correct way to carry out these exercises with the patient. Also, a physician demonstrating to her medical students how to acquire a blood sample from a patient for an arterial blood gas includes the preceptee in that same learning session. Numerous opportunities exist in which staff and other health team members continuously act as a learning resource within the context of the preceptorship experience.

Source of Preceptee Support

Staff acceptance and support are essential ingredients for a successful preceptorship. If staff do not accept and support preceptees, the road can be a long, uphill battle. In the practice setting, preceptees begin to use the various theories that they have learned in the familiarity of the classroom. Although preceptees learn different ways of dealing with nursing situations within the comfort of classroom and laboratory settings, it is in the unfamiliar and often daunting surroundings of the practice setting that they begin to acquire the ability to apply that knowledge to patient situations. Of particular significance, preceptees must learn to adapt and accommodate the idiosyncrasies of staff while going through the process. If staff members do not welcome and accept the preceptees, "this can become a formidable and not infrequently insurmountable challenge" (Myrick & Yonge, 2001, p. 466). Thus, the staff must fulfill their roles in the preceptorship experience and support and welcome the preceptees into the practice environment.

A supportive environment is one in which preceptees believe that they are appreciated as being a valid part of the health team. They achieve this sense of acceptance and support in a climate where staff value learning and show them respect, regardless of the level of expertise or experience with which they arrive on the unit. "The teacher has first of all to reveal, to take away the veil covering many students' intellectual life, and help them see that their own life experiences, their own insights and convictions, their own intuitions and formulations are worth serious attention (Nouwen, 1966, p. 61). Preceptees are supported by staff who are open to differences in others, who allow them the freedom to explore different experiences that contribute to their learning and experiential growth, who create a safe environment in which they can question and be questioned without fear of reprisal, and who foster "the development of each individual" (Reilly & Oermann, 1985, p. 77). When staff support preceptees, they will inevitably thrive in the practice setting. If, on the other hand, they are not supportive, then the preceptorship experience can become a nightmare for the preceptee.

· · · · · · · · · · · · · · · · · · ·

Box 3 - 8

Practical Information: Responsibilities as Support

Staff supports the preceptorship experience by:

- Promoting an environment that is accepting to the preceptee
- Collaborating with the preceptor and the faculty regarding the preceptor role
- Providing feedback to the preceptee regarding competencies
- Working with the preceptee, preceptor, and faculty, when required, to contribute to the performance evaluation of students

• The Education Players

Preceptees

The impetus or major reason for instituting preceptorship as an approach to clinical teaching is to provide students/novice nurses with the best possible experience in the real world of clinical and/or community practice. This goal is met by pairing novice or student nurses with expert nurses who can act as their role model and resource and who can be available to the preceptees immediately on a one-to-one basis as they carry out their nursing care and proceed through the learning process (Kaviani & Stillwell, 2000). As with the preceptor, the preceptees must be active players who contribute directly to the preceptorship experience success. Therefore, they assume various roles that are key to that success. Those roles follow.

Professional

The student or novice nurse's role as a preceptee is extremely important. It propels students or novice nurses into the professional domain of nursing practice, a context that requires them to behave professionally. Yet what exactly does being professional mean? Professionalism requires preceptees to display a demeanor and actions that reflect an unwavering adherence to the standards of nursing practice, to carry out nursing care safely and competently, and to demonstrate an ongoing

---

B o x   3 - 9

Practical Information: Responsibilities as a Professional

A preceptee acts as a professional by:

- Demonstrating a strong sense of commitment to his or her role in the preceptorship experience
- Adhering to ethical and nursing standards of practice
- Interacting with the preceptor, faculty, patients, families, colleagues, fellow students, and other members of the health team respectfully
- Being knowledgeable within his or her scope of practice as a student
- Reflecting prudent and careful judgment in clinical decision making

sense of commitment to the learning process. The preceptees' interactions with the preceptor, faculty, patients, their families, colleagues, fellow students, and other members of the health team illustrate the preceptees' commitment to professionalism. To be professional is to be knowledgeable (to the extent that is possible in the preceptee role) about nursing care and to be respectful of patients and coworkers. To be professional is to be ethical in practice, to be prudent or careful in clinical judgments, and to proceed in a way that is invariably considerate of the patient's well-being.

Reliable Learner/Student

Within the preceptorship experience, it is critical that preceptees be reliable/dependable. The preceptor should be able to count on the students or novice nurses to follow through with the various roles, responsibilities, and patient assignments that fit within their scope of practice. The preceptor must know that the preceptees will follow through when required to conduct particular requests, fulfill learning objectives, and complete nursing care safely and competently. For example, when responsible for patient care and required to administer medications, preceptees display reliability in how they proceed to organize and prepare for that particular care aspect. If preceptees consistently organize medications for administering in a timely fashion and are knowledgeable about the dosages, side effects, precautions, etc., the preceptor is confident in the preceptees' dependability in following through with that particular care aspect. In other words, although the preceptor is there to support and

---

B o x   3 - 1 0

Practical Information: Responsibilities as a Reliable
Learner/Student

The preceptee demonstrates reliability by:

- Following through on the various roles and patient assignments for which he or she is responsible
- Behaving in a consistent manner
- Maintaining organization in nursing care
- Being safe and competent in nursing actions

B o x   3 - 1 1

Practical Information: Responsibilities as an Accountable Participant

The preceptee should establish accountability by:

• Preparing for patient assignments
• Accepting responsibility for his or her own actions
• Contributing to learning experiences through his or her knowledge of the academic program and practice expectations and complying with those expectations in the completion of nursing care
• Being proactive in his or her interactions with the preceptor, staff, and other health team members

guide the preceptees through the preceptorship experience, the preceptor should not need to remind them to prepare medications or take the initiative in organizing facets of patient care. The preceptor derives confidence from the preceptees' actions.

Reliable learners assume responsibility for their own learning. Preceptees who routinely identify learning objectives, validate them with the preceptor, and then negotiate a timely and effective way to achieve them demonstrate initiative and reflect reliability. Also, by being proactive in discussing the daily objectives of nursing care and by exploring potential experiences in the practice setting that can further contribute to achieving learning objectives, preceptees show initiative and dependability in assuming responsibility for their learning.

Accountable Participant

Closely associated with the notion of reliability, preceptees must also be accountable. Although the role of preceptees within the preceptorship experience is primarily as learners in the practice setting, they are nevertheless expected to be both responsible and accountable for their own professional actions. Therefore, it is important that the preceptees are thoroughly prepared to assume patient assignments. For example, they should arrive on the unit having already explored the different aspects of assigned patients' particular conditions and contexts, so they can carry out nursing care safely and competently. Preceptees should (1) study the key nursing care and medical treatments for assigned patients, (2) thoroughly review the kinds of medications for which they will be responsible, and (3) consider the ramifications that the patient role has not only for their individual patients but also for the patient's family. Also, the preceptees should be prepared to address any questions that preceptors or other health team members may ask regarding their patient assignments.

Self-Evaluator

A true hallmark of success is the ability to be able to possess insight into one's own actions or performance. To achieve this self-awareness, preceptees must identify their strengths and recognize those areas of performance where they require additional assistance. Therefore, preceptors and preceptees must discuss performance on an ongoing basis. Such a process is often referred to as formative evaluation, because it provides preceptees with an opportunity to improve their performance and does not concern grading. However, for this process to be constructive, preceptees must communicate openly with preceptors and seek regular feedback for continuing improvement of their clinical performance. Also, they should be active participants in the evaluation process. Acting on the preceptor's feedback enables preceptees to continually improve their performance. Most important, if preceptees discover that they have a different perspective than the preceptor regarding performance, they must develop the ability and take the initiative to seek opportunities to engage in constructive dialogue or respectful discussion with the preceptor. Such

---

Box 3 - 12

Practical Information: Responsibilities as Self-Evaluator

The preceptee engages in self-evaluation by:

- Identifying areas of strength and recognizing areas of performance that require improvement
- Engaging (regularly) in discussion with the preceptor about his or her clinical performance
- Integrating preceptor feedback into his or her actions
- Keeping the lines of communication open between preceptee and preceptor at all times

a process will help to circumvent any miscommunication or misunder-standings that may potentially arise between preceptees and preceptors.

Faculty

Faculty members are pivotal to the success of the preceptorship experi-ence. They bring a wealth of substantive knowledge and key insights into understanding the teaching-learning process. Subsequently, they are an invaluable resource to both preceptors and preceptees. On one level, fac-ulty can be considered the preceptors of the preceptor (regarding the ped-agogic process). Because of their intrinsic involvement in the students' academic program and their direct input into the students' learning objectives, faculty are central in configuring the preceptorship experience so that it can adequately and effectively meet the students' capability lev-els. Although the preceptor brings a knowledge and expertise of clinical practice to preceptorship, faculty members bring the educational perspec-tive—both of which are *necessary* but neither of which is *sufficient* for its success. Moreover, professional practice would not survive without both the practice dimension *and* the theoretical or educational underpinnings that drive it. The preceptee needs theoretical preparation but must trans-late that theory within the nursing practice context. Thus, the working relationship between faculty and the preceptor is a key factor in how well the preceptorship plays out. Similar to the preceptor, preceptee, and staff, faculty assume various roles and responsibilities within the preceptor-ship experience.

Resource

Although the preceptor acts as a major support to the preceptee from a clinical practice perspective, faculty provide key educational support for *both* preceptor *and* preceptee. The preceptor must rely on faculty to guide the experience in the appropriate direction. Therefore, it is critical that faculty remain active participants in the entire process. Although it is accurate to assume that the preceptor and the student are foreground players in the preceptorship experience, faculty may be considered the background players with significant influence concerning how the expe-rience ensues.

To be an effective resource, it is particularly important that faculty are available and accessible to both the preceptor and the preceptee throughout the entire preceptorship experience trajectory. For example,

· · · · · · · · · · · · · · · · ·

┌───┐
| **B o x   3 - 1 3** |
| **Practical Information:** Responsibilities as Resource |
├───┤
| Faculty fulfill their role as resource to the preceptorship experience by: |
| • Acting as a major support to the preceptee and preceptor |
| • Being active participants in and contributors to the preceptorship experience |
| • Meeting with the preceptor in person |
| • Visiting the site of the preceptorship experience |
| • Making themselves available and accessible at all times throughout the preceptorship |
└───┘

faculty should stay physically connected to the unit in which the preceptorship is occurring if the setting is within commuting distance. They need to establish a pattern whereby they meet, on a one-on-one basis, with the preceptor at least one or more times throughout the entire preceptorship process. Meeting with the preceptor is especially important at the beginning of the preceptorship. Then, faculty must ensure that they remain connected via telephone and/or e-mail. Of equal significance, faculty must ensure that the preceptee is aware of their presence in the practice setting. Although the authors are not suggesting that faculty members interject themselves into the preceptorship relationship, it is extremely important that they at least strive to maintain a presence. That presence, in turn, implies and illustrates both the faculty's serious investment in the success of the preceptorship experience and the notion that they are available as required. This connection is critical to the success of the preceptorship experience.

Custodian of the Teaching-Learning Process

The unfolding of the teaching-learning process in the preceptorship experience lies directly within the faculty's purview. How well that process unfolds depends largely on faculty members' diligence to stay connected and be available to the preceptor and the preceptee as required. Faculty must ensure that the preceptorship experience meets the goals and objectives of the academic program and that the preceptor's expectations align with the overall learning objectives. Without faculty's input, a disconnec-

• • • • • • • • • • • • • • • • •

Box   3 - 1 4

Practical Information: Responsibilities as Custodian of the Teaching-Learning Process

Faculty act as custodian of the teaching-learning process by:

- Facilitating congruency between the preceptees' objectives and the preceptors' expectations
- Ensuring that the goals and objectives of the academic program are achieved
- Clarifying the educational perspective
- Consulting with the preceptor regarding the preceptee's patient assignments
- Maintaining open lines of communication between the practice and academic settings or practice and administration
- Creating opportunities that foster ongoing dialogue
- Discussing potential teaching strategies that can facilitate the preceptorship experience

tion between preceptor expectations and learner objectives may occur. Such disconnection can create havoc for both the preceptee and the preceptor and can result in an unfavorable experience for both. As custodian of the teaching-learning process, faculty must ensure clarity regarding the educational perspective, maintain open lines of communication between the practice and academic environments, and create opportunities that foster ongoing dialogue about the learning trajectory. The learning process, then, is optimal for all players involved, especially for the preceptee. Intrinsic to the faculty's role as custodian of the teaching-learning process is their ability to consult with the preceptor. For example, occasionally it may be necessary for faculty to advise the preceptor concerning the appropriate selection of patient assignments, the learning opportunities to which the preceptor should expose the preceptee, and increasing preceptee responsibilities within the context of his or her learning requirements. Faculty should take the initiative in connecting with the preceptor (eg, letting the preceptor know that they are available whenever required). This is not to suggest that faculty take the lead but that they make it clear that they are there when needed to provide input to all aspects of the teaching-learning process.

Evaluator

Aligned with their duties as custodians of the teaching-learning process and guardians of the orientation process, faculty serve as evaluators. They assume ultimate responsibility for the evaluation and final grading of the preceptees' performance. Faculty hold responsibility for the evaluation of preceptor performance and evaluation of the overall preceptorship experience. It is important that they provide ongoing feedback to the preceptors regarding their performance as clinical teachers, discuss potential clinical teaching strategies that preceptors may use, and provide input regarding the preceptees' performance. Whenever the preceptor or preceptee raises concerns about performance, it is important that faculty act on that feedback immediately. They should not allow it to go unchecked. As the old adage indicates, an ounce of prevention is worth a pound of cure. In other words, faculty should be proactive rather than reactive in their involvement in the evaluation process. Although they act as advisers to the preceptor, faculty also must give input to the preceptees regarding how best they can achieve their learning objectives and perform within the expectations of the academic program or agency. Therefore, it is essential that faculty ensure lines of communication are open among all players at all times.

• • • • • • • • • • • • • • • • • • • •

B o x   3 - 1 5

Practical Information: Responsibilities as Evaluator

Faculty's role as evaluator is critical to the success of the preceptorship experience; they fulfill their duties by:

- Assuming ultimate responsibility for the final evaluation and grading of the preceptees' clinical performance
- Seeking ongoing input from the preceptor regarding preceptee performance
- Providing feedback to the preceptor regarding his or her teaching performance
- Responding immediately to any concerns raised by the preceptors or preceptees
- Providing input to the preceptees concerning how best they can achieve their objectives

Another major aspect of the faculty evaluator role is their responsibility to assess the appropriateness of the unit on which the preceptorship is occuring. Is the overall atmosphere conducive to the teaching-learning process? Are staff members generally accepting of preceptees? Nothing is more discouraging to preceptees, particularly novice students, than to be viewed as strangers, ignored, or simply not supported when assigned to a particular unit. In fact, such an experience can be quite devastating. Also, if the preceptor who is assigned to the student is assuming the role because he or she is "required to" and not because he or she aspires to, the preceptee may have an unpleasant experience. In describing such an experience, a preceptee states, "I hated it, and I don't think it had anything to do with anything else but the fact that the preceptor didn't want to be a preceptor. It was hugely disappointing" (Myrick, 1998, p. 53). As another student stated when reflecting on the anxiety that occurred among her and her classmates when preparing for a preceptorship experience, "Our biggest fear was getting a grumpy preceptor, like somebody who was forced into doing it, who didn't want to do it, and just basically having to struggle through with this miserable person" (Myrick, 1998, p. 53). If faculty are diligent in evaluating the unit through site visits, interactions with the preceptor and the staff, and contact with the nurse unit manager, they will be able to ascertain whether difficulties such as the ones described are occurring. The decision may then be necessary to select a different unit on which to assign the student in the future.

Role Model

Like the preceptor is a role model for the preceptee, faculty members, in turn, are role models for both preceptor and preceptee. How faculty mem-

---

B o x 3 - 1 6

Practical Information: Responsibilities as Role Model

Faculty role model by:

- Being professional in their interactions with preceptees, preceptors, and staff
- Reflecting a sincerity of purpose
- Demonstrating a valuing of the perspectives of others
- Remaining open to other ways of thinking when approaching situations
- Being collaborative

bers conduct themselves is extremely important. For example, in their interactions with the preceptor, faculty must be professional, respectful, and focused on the success of the preceptorship experience. Therefore, it is particularly significant for faculty to reflect a sincerity of purpose in their interactions with those in the practice setting and to demonstrate a valuing of their perspectives and input. Although faculty are knowledgeable about the teaching-learning process, the academic program and the discipline of nursing, how they impart that knowledge reflects a sense of who they are as educators. Being open to other perspectives and ways of doing things is an excellent role model for collaboration, which can only contribute to the success of the preceptorship experience.

• Summary

The preceptorship experience involves a complex dynamic. The roles of preceptees, preceptors, faculty, and staff are multifaceted and are pivotal to the education of the future practitioner and leaders of the nursing profession. This chapter provides you with some preliminary discussion and insights into these key roles and responsibilities and reviews the contribution made by these various players to the preceptorship experience. The ensuing chapters further build on and enhance this discussion and thus provide you with additional insights, suggestions, and ideas that will assist and facilitate you in your preceptorship endeavor.

R E F E R E N C E S

Beckett, C., & Wall, M. (1985). Role of the clinical facilitator. *Nurse Education Today, 5,* 259–262.

Betz, C. (1985). Students in transition: Imitators of role models. *Journal of Nursing Education, 24,* 301–303.

Bidwell, A. S., & Brasler, M. L. (1989). Role modeling versus mentoring in nursing education. *IMAGE: Journal of Nursing Scholarship, 21,* 23–25.

Bizek, K., & Oermann, M. (1990). Study of educational experiences, support and job satisfaction among critical care nurse preceptors. *Heart & Lung, 19,* 439–444.

Concise Oxford Dictionary. (7th ed.) (1982). London: Oxford University Press.

Davis, E. (1993). Clinical role modeling: Uncovering hidden knowledge. *Journal of Advanced Nursing, 18,* 627–636.

Facione, N. C., & Facione, P. A. (1996). Externalizing the critical thinking in knowledge development and clinical judgment. *Nursing Outlook, 44,* 129–136.

Howie, J. (1988). The effective clinical: A role model. *Australian Journal of Advanced Nursing, 5*, 23–26.

Infante, M., Forbes, E., Houldin, A., & Nayler, M. (1989). A clinical teaching project: Examination of a clinical teaching model. *Journal of Professional Nursing, 5*, 132–139.

Kaviani, N., & Stillwell, Y. (2000). An evaluative study of clinical preceptorship. *Nurse Education Today, 33*, 31–34.

Myrick, F. (1998). *Preceptorship and critical thinking in nursing education.* Unpublished doctoral dissertation, University of Alberta, Edmonton, Alberta, Canada.

Myrick, F. (2002). Preceptorship and critical thinking in nursing education. *Journal of Nursing Education, 41*, 154–164.

Myrick, F., & Yonge, O. (2001). Creating a climate for critical thinking in the preceptorship experience. *Nurse Education Today, 21*, 461–467.

Nouwen, H. (1966). *Reaching out.* New York: Doubleday.

Reilly, D. E., & Oermann, M. H. (1985). *The clinical field. Its use in nursing education.* Norwalk, CT: Appleton-Century-Crofts.

Reilly, D. E., & Oermann, M. H. (1992). *Clinical teaching in nursing education* (2nd ed.). New York: National League for Nursing.

CHAPTER 4

The Preceptorship Focus

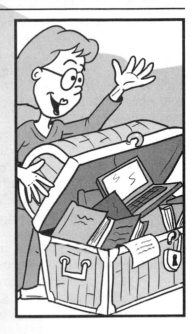

E ach participant in the preceptorship experience strives for success and hopes to achieve particular goals and objectives. Those goals and objectives are multifaceted and are generated from various perspectives, including those from the educational program teachers, practice agency administrators, preceptors, and preceptees.

• Educational Program Goals

In North America, preceptorship, as described in this textbook, was identified as a viable teaching method in the 1970s. As nurse educators became more involved in nursing education and developed nursing curricula based on broad concepts, such as health, man, and society, coupled with nursing frameworks based on nursing theorists, such as Roy, Orem, Watson, Henderson, and so forth, a new legitimacy to the profession and discipline of nursing evolved. At the same time, there was a shift in nursing education from hospital-based programs to colleges and universities.

This shift resulted in increased numbers of students having access to academic programs that were increasingly taught by teachers who not only had to teach in the clinical areas but also had to prove their worth in academic settings through research and knowledge dissemination. Such expectations were challenging because nursing is a practice discipline and, as such, demands that educators keep abreast of the latest clinical innovations. To assist the educator in retaining clinical expertise, strategies such as clinical joint and adjunct appointments emerged. The longer the teacher was in an institution, such as a university, the less likely he or she was to teach in the clinical area because of the competing demands generated by the need to conduct research and the excessive time required for clinical teaching (Myrick, 1991). Furthermore, it was easier to hire temporary staff for clinical teaching versus a classroom setting. Unfortunately, the longer the educators did not teach in the clinical area, the less likely they were inclined to do so, given the rapid changes in care delivery systems resulting from health system restructuring and the escalation of health care technology. In other words, they simply lost their comfort and confidence in clinical teaching.

Preceptorship programs filled a void for teachers who found themselves stretched in multiple directions. However, such programs also served to meet the needs of preceptors and students as well. In the 1970s in North America, more nurses in the workforce began identifying themselves as professionals with a distinct body of knowledge. They believed that they had the expertise to be preceptors and to teach peers, students, and patients in hospital and community settings. At the same time, teachers in the educational institutions were intent on designing preceptorship programs that were ethical, were professional, and would enhance student learning and development. In other words, nursing education was to be shared with the service-delivery sector. This meant that students would be enrolled in courses, usually in the final year of their programs, that reflected course objectives embracing ethical and legal practice, the growing body of nursing knowledge, guidelines on being a team member in a particular area of nursing, and so forth. Daily evaluation became the jurisdiction of the preceptor, with the overall course evaluations remaining under the auspices of the nurse educator. Students were required to adhere to the conduct regulations for both the educational institution and the standards for professional nursing practice.

Thus, the goals for preceptorship programs from the educational perspective evolved to ensure that current students are prepared for a preceptorship experience. Readiness is determined through adequate clinical and theoretical preparation, specific educational interventions (such as learning how to manage conflict) (Yonge, Krahn, Trojan, & Reid,

1997), faculty assessment of student skills and attitudes, and a certain academic standing, particularly for students who are accessing international practica. Readiness is occasionally difficult to ascertain from both the student's and the teacher's perspective. Occasionally, students will commence a preceptorship program and discover, much to their dismay, that it is the wrong site for them or that it is simply the wrong time for them to be participating in a preceptorship program (Yonge, Myrick & Haase, 2002). A small number of students need the support of their peers in a clinical teaching group or an experienced clinical teacher in their final program year.

Clinical and community sites for preceptorship are usually chosen through the collaboration of educators, administrators, and faculty. Because various nursing educational institutions may be competing for a limited number of practica in certain sites, tensions and disappointments can occur. Students are reminded that a choice of a practicum site is a privilege and not a right. At times, some students may try to circumvent the process by obtaining their own practicum, particularly if they have friends or relatives working in a highly valued clinical or practice area, such as an intensive care setting or emergency department. Educators remain steadfast in their belief that regardless of the practicum in a selected site, students must fulfill the learning objectives of the preceptorship program relative to the course in which the preceptorship is associated. The first priority is that students have the ability to achieve the learning objectives of the course taught through the preceptorship method (see Appendix B).

Preceptorship can be a freeing and affirming experience. Students may experience the following for the first time: rotating shifts, access to highly specialized interventions, work situations demanding quick decision making and priority setting, and challenges in managing complex situations. When students feel that they are supported throughout the preceptorship experience, they usually have increased competence and confidence. This is illustrated in the story of Jean who had a 6-week preceptorship in northern Canada. She worked in an outpost nursing station with an experienced preceptor. The patients were indigenous to the area and had a culture in which she was the stranger and the person of minority status. As she began to understand her role in the community and the patients' behaviors, she became more effective in meeting their health care needs. When she returned to southern Canada and had a debriefing interview with a faculty member, she stated that she now knew that she truly wanted to be a nurse. She elaborated that as a result of the preceptorship experience, she had acquired the maturity and the depth required to be a nurse. When questioned why she had come to that realization, she stated that it was the result of having been out of her comfort zone and discovering that she could function in situations that were initially "way over her head." The feedback and acknowledgment she received from her preceptor and the community also affirmed that she wanted to be a nurse. She thanked the faculty member for having facilitated the preceptorship experience and, in her words, for having "changed her life." Jean may have had the same reaction had she completed a preceptorship experience in a local acute care facility. However, by living away from home and being an outsider to a community in a culture where she was in the minority and relying on a small support base, she had placed herself in a vulnerable position and discovered that she not only had the skills and ability to contribute to the community in a professional nursing capacity but that she also could flourish in the process.

Ultimately, the goal for all students is to provide professional, ethical, and safe nursing care. To do so, they must work with a preceptor who also possesses those characteristics. One possible way of acknowledging those values is to institute a formal process in which educational institutions integrate the experience of the preceptor role as a criterion for admission into postgraduate programs. Such a policy would acknowledge the professional work of preceptorship and, although the preceptor may not have taught a formal course to the preceptee, he or she nevertheless can be recognized for having used the principles of teaching and learning.

• Goals of Administrators in Health Care Agencies

Before the movement of nursing education out of the hospital-based programs, students staffed the hospital for some period of their training. With the closure of the hospital training programs, administrators quickly lost low-paid student workers and new graduates from the hospital-based program. The emergence of preceptorship meant that students were socialized into the hospital or other health care agency settings, were preceptored one-on-one, and perhaps even mentored, and because of this close teaching-learning relationship, they returned to their preceptorship site to seek employment. Administrators had the privilege of observing students in the preceptorship practicum and could make a better hiring decision. If students were then employed by the agency in the same area as their preceptorship practicum, their orientation time was decreased. Administrators soon saw the benefits of facilitating preceptorship experiences.

However, there have been conflicts emanating from administration's expectations. Administration may assign a double patient workload to a preceptor because he or she is assigned a preceptee. The administrator assumes that a student means an extra set of hands. Throughout the preceptorship experience, if a preceptor calls in ill, an administrator is likely to assign the student the preceptor's usual duties, stating that there is no need to hire extra staff, believing that the student knows what he or she is doing. In these situations, a student may be told to consult any staff member if he or she has questions or concerns, and, in doing so, the teaching role of the preceptor is not acknowledged.

Regardless of these conflicts, administrators usually welcome the opportunity to precept students. The outcomes for administrators are increased retention of staff, particularly if preceptors are appropriately acknowledged for their work; recruitment of preceptees as potential staff; and contribution to a more professional working environment. The latter occurs when staff members model professional behaviors. Preceptees bring with them an enthusiasm for the profession, ongoing questions, and a strong work ethic. Their vitality ultimately infects other staff.

If recruitment to a clinical or community site is an issue, administrators may offer incentives to preceptees. Such incentives range from living accommodations and food, to an honorarium, to future employment. Preceptees may hear promises of educational development opportunities, such as postgraduate work. In fact, there have been occasions when an administrator has informed potential preceptees that they can only obtain a preceptorship experience if they, in turn, seek employment in that agency for a certain length of time. Such a proposition usually poses a challenge for the preceptees if they are unsure where they will seek employment or in which area they would like to begin their careers.

• Preceptors' and Preceptees' Goals

Preceptorship is a form of structured teaching, and learning for preceptees is the most obvious goal and most always identified as the core of the experience. Preceptors possess a unique body of knowledge, and, usually, this knowledge can be accessed only through this type of program. For example, a small clinical area, such as a liver transplant unit, can only accommodate 1 or 2 students, as opposed to the traditional 8- to 10-student clinical group. Preceptorships provide solutions to increased pressures in health care and one of these pressures involves the accom-

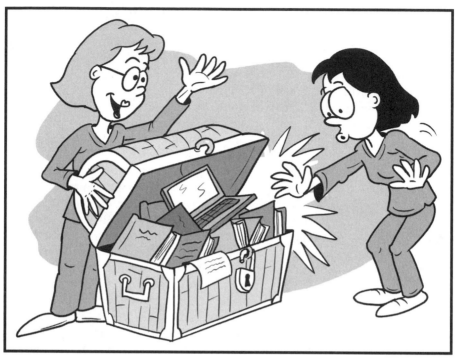

Preceptorship allows preceptors to share their unique treasures of knowledge and experience.

modation of large numbers of learners (Hill, Wolf, Bossetti, & Saddanm, 1999; Smith, McAllister, & Snype-Crawford, 2001).

Nevertheless, there is a hidden workload in precepting. Preceptors are volunteers and organize their workload to effectively accommodate learners, and, by doing so, they contribute not only to their profession but also to the overall agency climate. Preceptors have been asked why they do what they do and if they want to be rewarded for this. In a research article examining the question of rewards, 295 preceptors responded and stated that they did not want to be rewarded but wanted to be acknowledged (Yonge, 1995). They wanted sufficient time to spend with students so they could feel rewarded by seeing the results of their efforts, that is, student growth (Hill et al., 1999; Nolan, Reser, Owens, & Tollefson, 1999). They also reported that they view nonmonetary rewards to be the most rewarding (Greenburg, Colombrano, DeBlasio, Dolan, & Rich, 2001; Hill et al. 1999). Peceptors noted that they also preceptored for personal reasons. In other words, they assumed the role for professional development and job enrichment, which promoted a sense of job satisfaction (Jones, Murtaugh, Durkin, Bolden, & Majewski, 2000; Smith et al., 2001). Although there are agencies that provide preceptors with financial remuneration for assuming their role, most acknowledge preceptors through educational gifts, including time to attend workshops, or small tokens, such as pens and pins. Yonge (1995) found that the most important acknowledgment was a personal detailed letter sent to the preceptor and administration. The letter could then be used for the staff member's performance appraisal.

The role of the preceptor also depends on the needs of the educational institution, administration, and preceptee. Preceptors question their role (Andrews & Wallis, 1999; Dyson, 1999) and desire to know the boundaries and scope of their role. Designers of preceptorship programs, particularly those without a background in adult education, may not understand why preceptors must have defined roles. An assumption underlying this lack of understanding is the belief that one simply teaches another what he or she knows. On the surface, this may be the case, but years of experience and education cannot simply be taught verbally in short interactions or nonverbally through role modeling. Therefore, it is not surprising that preceptors question how much responsibility, autonomy, or power they can expect in their particular role. They also want to know the expectations of their peers, the administration, external agencies, and preceptees. For example, they want to know what they should do if the preceptee is unsafe and how they should manage such a preceptee. In the evaluation, they question if they are limited to giving feedback or if they are expected to grade a preceptee. If the preceptee has an excessive number of days away because of illness or unexplained absences, they want to know who is responsible for tracking the time or following up with the preceptee. What about the times when the preceptee behaves unethically, such as using undue force and aggression with the patient? The preceptor might give feedback to the preceptee about this behavior, but the preceptor questions how the broken trust will be repaired between the preceptee and preceptor. There are also circumstances in which a preceptee requests an uncommon experience, such as accompanying the preceptor on an emergency medical evacuation. What if the airplane should crash during the evacuation: will the preceptor be liable if the preceptee is harmed or killed? If the preceptee engages in a criminal act, such as stealing medications from a patient, preceptors want to know their obligations and reporting lines. They want to know if they have to provide documentation on the preceptee's behaviors and who will be reading that documentation. If an act is serious, they question if they will be involved in hearings or external investigations.

As well, preceptors teach many different levels of preceptees, from new staff to undergraduate students to graduate students, and it is possible to teach students from several disciplines. For example, a preceptor working in an intensive care area may have nursing, medical, emergency medical technicians, or respiratory technician students. Students may also come from different programs locally, nationally, or internationally. Furthermore, each preceptee brings with him or her a body of knowledge based on his or her experiences and learning objectives.

There may be instances when a preceptee may be more proficient than the preceptor. Such a situation is illustrated in the following example. Kristin was a fourth-year nursing student who selected a preceptorship rotation in another country so she could travel after she completed the rotation. She was placed in a pediatric department. Shortly before her arrival, the staff members were instructed that they would be starting all the IV lines. Until that time, a special IV team managed all IVs. The staff members were reticent about starting IVs on the patients because they believed that they no longer possessed that skill and did not want to be the "givers of pain" to children. The staff members were told they had no choice and were offered inservices to upgrade their skills. One day was designated for the changeover, and this day happened to be Kristin's first day on rotation. Her preceptor was to start two IVs, and as she was about to do the first one, she blanched and said she could not do it. Kristin, observing the anxiety in her preceptor, stated that she would be glad to do it. The preceptor was incredulous. Kristin reassured her and informed the preceptor that she was an emergency medical technician before she entered nursing and was highly proficient in starting IVs under stressful conditions. The preceptor turned over the equipment to Kristin, and the procedure was completed efficiently. The preceptor started the second IV with Kristin observing. As the rotation progressed, Kristin worked with her preceptor and the other staff, helping them develop confidence in starting IVs. At the termination of the rotation, the staff gave Kristin a personalized IV set, spray painted with gold. Kristin thanked everyone for everything she had learned in the rotation, particularly her preceptor, who taught her how to communicate with parents and siblings of children who were gravely ill. She acknowledged that she had been happy to share her ability to start IVs but this was simply one skill in an area that was rich with many and varied skills and experience.

Looking at the preceptor role through the eyes of students, Grey and Smith (2000) researched students' perceptions of what made a preceptor effective. The students believed that preceptors should be friendly, approachable, professional, organized, knowledgeable, realistic, and respected by other team members. The last point is important. Although preceptors are assigned to the role, how others view them and what others perceive their role to be inevitably affect the quality of teaching for the student. If others respect the preceptor, the preceptee feels more confident in the preceptor's abilities.

Nolan et al. (1999) state that preceptors must be committed to their role. While this may sound like a straightforward assertion, in practice preceptors have initially committed to the role only to find that they no longer want or can have that responsibility. When this happens, it is not uncommon for other team members step in and assume that role.

Such an occurrence is illustrated by Sara's story. Sara worked on a busy surgical unit. She was a highly skilled nurse and was happy to accept a nursing student. The experience was positive, and the following year, she was again approached and asked if she would be a preceptor. She readily agreed. The student started at the beginning of the month and within 1 week, Sara's grandmother died. The others on the team preceptored her student. She returned from the funeral, worked 2 weeks, and was then notified that her grandfather had committed suicide. He had been severely depressed after losing his wife of 55 years. Sara attended the funeral. When she returned to work, she informed the charge nurse that she no longer wished to continue with the preceptorship arrangement. She stated that she was grieving and did not have the energy to be a preceptor. Three of her peers volunteered to form a preceptor team for the student.

As in Sara's case, more than one staff member may be the preceptor for the preceptee. If agencies employ a high number of part-time staff, it is common for two preceptors to be assigned to one preceptee. It is a form of job sharing. Most preceptees appreciate this arrangement if the two preceptors have similar teaching styles and respect each other's abilities. However, occasionally a preceptee will be assigned to a specialized team or program, such as an inner-city program for women in poverty or a northern nursing station. All team members must be committed to teaching the preceptee, and usually the only behavior that needs negotiation is evaluation of the preceptee. This responsibility typically falls to the person who is in charge of the team, but ultimately everyone contributes to the final evaluation.

The role is not static for the preceptor or preceptee. The preceptee, regardless of whether a student or new staff member, is in the transition process. This transition has been termed as iterative, interactive, and dynamic (Godinez, Schweiger, Gruver, & Ryan, 1999). Specific skills to learn can be targeted, and broader skills, such as organization, priority setting, and critical thinking, are fostered. The preceptor too is in transition: developing teaching, communication, and management skills. These skills can apply to other settings and circumstances.

• Orientation

The first week of work in the agency can and does influence the preceptees' perceptions for the entire rotation. The challenge for the preceptor is to orient the preceptee actively and effectively (Bumgarner & Biggerstaff, 2000). Orientation can assume many forms, from show and tell, treasure hunts, and use of self-directed modules (Holtzman, 1999) to specific and well-defined activities (Schulz & DiSanto, 1999). Orientation is usually based on the available time and needs of the preceptor and preceptee. Bumgarner and Biggerstaff (2000) decided to develop a patient-focused program. They asked, if staff members had a patient-focused pathway, what specific skills would the preceptor and preceptee need? The skills were identified, and then the preceptor taught these skills to the preceptee. On completion of the pathway pilot application, they reported that there was greater job satisfaction, an increase in the quality of patient care, and notable staff retention. They did not include the means to measure these outcomes; however, they captured the central focus of preceptorship, which is patient care. Preceptors and preceptees must continually remind themselves that they are teaching and learning for the distinct purpose of providing safe and ethical patient care. If preceptors begin orientation of preceptees with this mandate, preceptees will have the right focus.

Orientation to an agency may occur at numerous levels. There may be a general orientation for all staff levels, a specific orientation for a program, and then a preceptor-provided orientation. Coordinators of student preceptorship programs must specifically request that agencies provide an orientation for students that is broader than the one provided by the preceptor. This level of orientation is often neglected for the student and yet is needed for them to understand the agency landscape.

Frequently, there are instances in which the orientation does not occur in the first few shifts. A preceptee may arrive in the agency only to find that it is frenetic. Therefore, it is important that the preceptor communicate to the preceptee what he or she can do to assist and to reassure him or her that he or she is welcome. Terry's story illustrates this point. Terry arrived at 0630 hours to review the charts before meeting his preceptor at 0700 hours for report on his intensive care rotation. At 0655 hours, a code was called, only to be followed by another code at 0730 hours. The preceptor directed Terry to care for patients in the coronary observation room, which meant working with another staff member. Terry worked in the observation room for two shifts before his preceptor had time to orient him to the unit. Hopefully, this case is unusual. The best opportunity to provide orientation is when there is sufficient time for the preceptor to teach and for the preceptee to ask questions. If an agency is quiet on nights, then that might be the best time for a preceptee to begin a rotation. Preceptees also must read policy and procedure manuals and related literature. Sometimes preceptees will visit the agency before the rotation to determine how they should prepare for the orientation.

• Evaluation

Evaluation of preceptees' clinical performance is a continuing issue for educators, as well as preceptors. Neary (2000, 2001) used a simple survey with three open-ended questions and found that preceptors were confused about their responsibilities in the evaluation process. Evaluation is typically guided by some type of teacher-designed tool and may include student self-evaluation and evaluative comments from other staff members. The evaluation tools for clinical work are typically not standardized, nor have they been tested for reliability or validity. Preceptors use variations of these tools.

Part of the difficulty in evaluation relates to how preceptors evaluate preceptees in a changing clinical environment (Dumas, Villeneuve, & Chevrier, 2000). As the environment changes, so does the preceptee. There is an expectation that the preceptee will become more independent with time and practice. If a preceptee is not progressing or is regressing, the preceptor becomes concerned. The preceptor's perception of the preceptee's work should be checked initially with the preceptee.

There are two models of evaluation published in the nursing research literature. Neary (2001) developed the Progressive Assessment Model of Evaluation, a complex model that would be exceedingly challenging to apply, and Bevis and Watson (1989/2000) developed the Interpretive Criticism Model of Educational Connoisseurship, a more user-friendly model than the one developed by Neary, but the authors admit this one is incomplete. More research is needed in this area.

The first step in evaluation is asking what is to be evaluated and then how the preceptor is to do this. In a survey of 295 preceptors, 28.8% stated that they were taught to evaluate nursing students (Yonge et al., 1997). It was not known from the survey results what was taught to the preceptors. The preceptee should be evaluated against program objectives. If the preceptee is a student, it is helpful for the preceptor to have a competency list documenting what the student has learned before arriving at the agency. It is important to note that although a competency may have been taught in the classroom, the student may not have had the opportunity or may have had a limited opportunity to master it. Therefore, the preceptee and preceptor must carefully review the competency list, and the preceptee must clearly identify his or her learning goals (Elliott, 2002). If an evaluation form is used as part of the preceptorship program, it should be reviewed at the beginning of the rotation. Both the preceptor and the preceptee must be aware of the standards and expectations for evaluation. Some preceptors review the criteria for evaluation of a preceptorship program on a daily basis, whereas others may prefer to wait until a midway or end point.

There is tension associated with the evaluation process, even if the evaluation is glowing. Part of that tension relates to the subjectivity and power of the evaluator, previous experiences with evaluation, and a fear of the unknown. Some preceptors prefer a formal method of evaluation, whereby they keep a journal of the student's behaviors and then write an evaluation with anecdotes. However, most prefer providing ongoing verbal feedback as needed and then completing a final informal evaluation. This results, in part, in the extra work of writing an evaluation, but it is also foreign to preceptors. Unlike educators, preceptors are not used to this activity.

The most challenging evaluation is one in which the preceptee demonstrates a poor performance level. If the preceptee is a student, the preceptor may have to recommend the faculty to fail the student; if the preceptee is in an orientation program, contract termination may be warranted. A situation that is most daunting is one in which the preceptee does not perceive that he or she has a poor performance level. This preceptee is unsafe.

• Summary

In summary, this chapter focuses on the goals of preceptorship from the view of the educators, administrators, preceptors, and preceptees. Preceptorship programs assist all parties in meeting their goals in ways that traditional programs cannot provide to the numbers of students in a clinical group and within the ever-changing structures in health care. Through preceptorship programs, preceptors and preceptees have had to assume more responsibility for professional education and, in turn, contribute to the professional nature of the workplace (see Box 4-1).

Box 4-1. Goals and Objectives of Preceptorship

- The goal for the educational institution is to prepare the preceptees for the preceptorship experience so that they can meet the course objectives in giving safe and ethical care and gain confidence and competence.
- Goals for administrators are recruitment and promotion of a professional work environment.
- A goal for both preceptors and preceptees is the fostering of a teaching-learning relationship, with both experiencing a change in behavior.
- Preceptors want and must know their role.
- Preceptors must be acknowledged for their work.
- Orientation is fundamental to the preceptorship process. A patient-focused orientation is core to the profession.
- Evaluation is a challenge for preceptors because of inadequate preparation, dynamic changing behaviors of the environment, and the use of tools that are not reliable or valid.

R E F E R E N C E S

Andrews, M., & Wallis, M. (1999). Mentorship in nursing: A literature review. *Integrative Literature Reviews and Meta-Analyses, 29,* 201–207.

Bevis, E., & Watson, J. (1989/2000). *Toward a caring curriculum: A new pedagogy for nursing.* New York: National League for Nursing.

Bumgarner, S. D., & Biggerstaff, G. H. (2000). A patient-centered approach to nurse orientation. *Journal of Nurse in Staff Development, 16,* 249–256.

Dumas, L., Villeneuve, J., & Chevrier, J. (2000). A tool to evaluate how to learn from experience in clinical settings. *Journal of Nursing Education, 39,* 251–258.

Dyson, L. (1999). The role of the lecturer in the preceptor model of clinical teaching. *Nursing Praxis in New Zealand, 16,* 16–24.

Elliott, M. (2002). The clinical environment: A source of stress for undergraduate nurses. *Australian Journal of Advanced Nursing, 20,* 34–38.

Godinez, G., Schweiger, J., Gruver, J., & Ryan, P. (1999). Role transition from graduate to staff nurse: A qualitative analysis. *Journal of Nurses in Staff Development, 15,* 97–110.

Greenberg, M., Colombraro, G., DeBlasio, J., Dolan, J., & Rich, E. (2001). Rewarding preceptors: A cost-effective model. *Nurse Educator, 26,* 114–116.

Grey, M. A., & Smith, L. (2000). The qualities of an effective mentor from the student nurse's perspective: Findings from a longitudinal qualitative study. *Journal of Advanced Nursing, 32*, 1542–1549.

Hill, N., Wolf, K. N., Bossetti, B., & Saddanm A. (1999). Preceptor appraisals of rewards and student preparedness in the clinical setting. *Journal of Allied Health, 28*, 86–90.

Holtzman, G. (1999). The development of a self-directed module for orientation of nursing students to multiple inpatient clinical sites. *Journal of Nursing Education, 38*, 380–381.

Jones, B., Murtaugh, M., Durkin, Z. A., Bolden, M. C., & Majewski, T. (2000). Clinical education in two-year colleges: Cost-benefit issues. *Journal of Allied Health, 29*, 109–113.

Myrick, F. (1991). The plight of clinical teaching in baccalaureate nursing education. *Journal of Nursing Education, 30*, 44–46.

Neary, M. (2000). Supporting students' learning and professional development through the process of continuous assessment and mentorship. *Nurse Education Today, 20*, 463–474.

Neary, M. (2001). Responsive assessment: Assessing student nurses' clinical competence. *Nurse Education Today, 21*, 3–17.

Nolan, C., Reser, P., Owens, J., & Tollefson, J. (1999). An exploration of the preceptor role: Preceptors' perceptions of benefits, rewards, supports and commitment to the preceptor role. *Journal of Advanced Nursing, 29*, 506–514.

Schulz, K. E., & DiSanto, K. (1999). Investing in the future—an OR orientation program for nursing students. *AORN Journal, 69*, 635, 637–638.

Smith, L. S., McAllister, L. E., & Snype-Crawford, C. (2001). Mentoring benefits and issues for public health nurses. *Public Health Nursing, 18*, 101–107.

Yonge, O. (1995). Acknowledging preceptors: Not an easy task. *The Journal of Continuing Education in Nursing, 26*, 150–157.

Yonge, O., Krahn, H., Trojan, L., & Reid, D. (1997). Through the eyes of the preceptors. *Canadian Journal of Nursing Administration, 12*, 65–85.

Yonge, O., Myrick, F., & Haase, M. (2002). Student nurse stress in the preceptorship experience. *Nurse Educator, 27*(2), 84–88.

PART II

Process

The Preceptor as "Teacher"

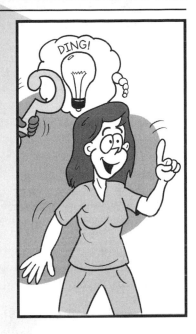

Good teaching cannot be reduced to technique; good teaching comes from the identity and integrity of the teacher.

Palmer, 1998, p. 10

Teaching by any standard is not a trivial proposition. It is a complex phenomenon from several perspectives: the ability to recognize that inherent complexity contributes to a successful outcome in the teaching-learning process. Teaching is a multidimensional process. Often, it can be quite demanding. Yet, it can be an eminently rewarding experience. Teaching is not, as one might assume, only about imparting one's knowledge and expertise to others. It is about motivating others to want to change through the acquisition of new knowledge. The effective teacher possesses the capacity to relay knowledge to learners so that it transforms their thinking and behavior. Effective teachers consider not only the subject matter or knowledge with which they are required to engage learners but also the recipients of that knowledge and how their actions as teachers affect individual learning, thinking, and behavior.

The role of teacher within the context of the preceptorship experience is no less complex. In this chapter, we provide several ideas and
strategies that will enhance your ability to teach successfully. A key factor to that success is your ability to create a climate in which preceptees
cannot only survive but also thrive in their learning and grow as professionals. Integral to that climate is your individual approach to the teaching-learning process. How you interact with and behave toward your
preceptee is critical. "Students must be led gently into the active role of
discussing, dialoguing, and problem solving" (Myrick & Yonge, 2001, p.
461). Preceptees are extremely sensitive to how respectfully you respond
to their comments, and they pick up on your nonverbal cues. When you
genuinely work with, value, and support them, you create an atmosphere of trust and acceptance; that atmosphere contributes to a positive
learning environment in which preceptees feel safe enough to question
and be questioned. Such an environment affords them a sense of security, which, in turn, contributes to their development as confident and
competent practitioners. Being mindful of the effect of your behavior and
approach with your preceptee will help provide a positive preceptorship
experience.

Teaching may not only be about technique but may also be about
possessing the relevant skills that will allow you to focus on various
dimensions of the teaching-learning process that are involved in the preceptorship experience. To facilitate your teaching, the following are discussed: selection of appropriate patient assignments, strategies to help
you promote your preceptees' ability to think critically, ways to foster preceptee autonomy, other teaching-learning strategies that will assist you
throughout the preceptorship experience, and relevant evaluation techniques.

• Selection of Appropriate Patient Assignments

Regardless of the level of the preceptees to whom you are assigned, you
will need to consistently judge the nature of their patient assignments.
Specifically, you will need to consider patient acuity, the complexity of the
patient's medical condition, and the requisite nursing care that is
involved. To guide you, there are several factors to consider. These include
the preceptees' learning objectives, your knowledge of the preceptees' previous clinical/practice experience, discussions with the preceptees, and
your connection with faculty.

The Preceptees' Learning Objectives

The preceptees' learning objectives provide you with a snapshot of the preceptees' specific expectations and reflect the academic requirements that will guide you in shaping the preceptorship experience toward the preceptees' learning needs. For example, a preceptee who is at the end of the fourth year usually will be able to assume a more complex patient assignment than the preceptee who is just beginning the year. As a rule of thumb, patient assignments must be congruent with the level of knowledge and practice experience of the individual preceptee. Even preceptees who are in the same year may present differently; that is, whereas one preceptee at a particular level is highly motivated, competent, and confident, another preceptee at the same level may be somewhat complacent, reluctant to seek new experiences, and insecure about performance. Such differences can be related to various factors that include, but are not limited to, the preceptees' individual capabilities, the quality of their previous practical experiences or lack thereof, and their own level of self-confidence. Normally, the preceptees' learning objectives are so specific that it is clear what types of experiences they will need to achieve those goals during the course of the preceptorship program (see Box 5-1).

B o x   5 - 1

Practical Information: Sample Learning Objectives

In conducting their nursing care, preceptees will be able to:

- Use multiple sources of information that contribute to the nursing care of their assigned patients
- Clearly delineate specific objectives for nursing care
- Prioritize appropriately and effectively
- Conduct nursing care safely and competently
- Demonstrate effective use of verbal and nonverbal communication skills
- Cooperate with peers, faculty, and health care team members
- Use the process and products of research to enhance clinical practice
- Assume responsibility for their own learning and competency; for example, readily and graciously accept guidance and supervision in the practice of their nursing care

The Preceptees' Previous Experience

A second tool at your disposal to help guide you in the selection of patient assignments is your knowledge or awareness of the preceptees' previous experience regarding their clinical or community practice. At the beginning of the preceptorship experience, it is critical that you acquire not only the preceptees' learning and program objectives but also a summary, preferably written, of their previous practica experiences and the specific skills they have mastered. Without this background information, it will be extremely challenging for you to make the appropriate choices for patient assignments. Unfortunately, there may be occasions when the preceptee will arrive on your unit without these important details. Subsequently, if such a situation occurs, it is within your right as preceptor to request that the preceptee provide you with this information as soon as possible. Otherwise, tensions can develop that otherwise could have been easily prevented or circumvented by this simple action. For example, if you are not in possession of this background information regarding the preceptees' previous experience, you may assume that they are capable of being assigned to a more complex patient assignment. In assigning such a patient without knowing this key detail, you discover that the preceptee flounders, which can create unease between you, your preceptee, and the patient. Therefore, it is not reasonable for you to be expected to commence the preceptorship experience without this significant information. In fact, it is essential for you to have this information in your hands before beginning the preceptorship experience (see Appendix C).

Discussions With the Preceptees

In addition to the preceptees' learning objectives and summary description of their previous practica experiences, it is important that you discuss patient selection with the preceptees. Preceptees' input into their learning is critical not only to the success of the preceptorship experience but also to their individual advancement as beginning nurses. Although ostensibly they may be neophytes to the unit on which you are preceptor, preceptees bring with them an abundance of life experiences that you must value. Some neophyte preceptees may have had other careers before entering the nursing profession or may have already completed a university degree external to nursing. Many preceptees may come to the preceptorship experience with a knowledge and wisdom that belies their neophyte role within nursing. Therefore, they must at least be respected. They must be treated as responsible adults who are accountable for their own actions. Thus, their input into their patient assignments would be entirely appropriate. However, this does not preclude your role in guiding their thinking. Occasionally, that guidance may mean that you will not always agree on particular selections. However, in that event, you can reach a reasonable decision through open, honest, and respectful dialogue between you and your preceptee. Traditionally, it has been the practice in the nursing profession that beginning students were consistently given direction in their experiences. In other words, they were told what to do, when to do it, and how to do it. Seldom were they afforded the opportunity to provide input into their own learning. This approach to clinical teaching created an atmosphere of subservience, which is diametrically opposed to the promotion of autonomy and critical thinking and the development of practical wisdom, all of which are essential qualities for professional practice and indicative of a competent and confident nurse. If preceptees are to develop their confidence, they will do so much more readily if you treat them with respect and if you involve them in decision making. By treating them as equal partners in the preceptorship experience, you send the message that you have confidence in their capability, and they, in turn, will strive to meet your expectations. They will feel valued and respected and will reflect this in their level of confidence. As one preceptor observed, "They [preceptees] are like a flower. They just open up" (Myrick, 1998, p. 76).

Connecting With the Faculty

If the preceptee is a student, a final tool in your repertoire for selecting appropriate patient assignments is your connection with the faculty member who is responsible for the academic course in which the student is enrolled. It is important that you and the particular faculty member develop a rapport that supports one another and in which the lines of communication are open and clear. If possible, connect with the faculty member before commencing the preceptorship experience. Ideally, it would be appropriate for you to meet with the faculty member and the preceptee together to clarify any questions or concerns that you may have regarding the preceptee's learning/program objectives or previous clinical experiences. By connecting face-to-face, it is much easier to ensure that you are all on the same page regarding the kind of experience required for the preceptee within the context of the preceptorship program. It is also an opportunity for the three of you to begin to develop a working relationship, become familiar with each other's communication and working styles, and clarify any questions or concerns that you may have. Once you have made that connection, you will be less reluctant to call on the faculty member if you require any feedback concerning patient assignments or if you have any questions related to the teaching-learning process. If it is not possible to meet face-to-face, then it would be appropriate to connect with one another by telephone or e-mail. The important point to remember is that you must connect directly with the faculty member who is involved in the preceptee's program. Ordinarily, it is the faculty member's responsibility to make that first connection. However, that does not preclude you from doing so should you wish.

• Strategies to Promote Critical Thinking

It is fair to say that the term *critical thinking* has become the buzzword of the past several decades, particularly in university education. The term has become most closely associated with the baccalaureate-prepared nurse. What exactly does critical thinking suggest? According to Facione and Facione (1996), critical thinking refers to "a nonlinear, recursive process in which a person forms a judgment about what to believe or what to do in a given context" (p. 131). In other words, it is a process in which the individual, in this case the preceptee, can deal with a situation by considering all aspects of that particular situation and subsequently reaching a reasonable understanding of what is required under those circumstances. From there, you can guide preceptees in their actions. Critical thinking is about being open to many possibilities and willing to think about situations from different vantage points. According to a popular phrase, critical thinking is about thinking outside the box. In practice, it is about always making the patient the focal point in each situation and considering the multidimensional context of patients and their families. Because a patient is always involved, as health professionals we should remember that the patient role is only one small dimension of who the individual is. Outside of that role, the patient may be a mother, father, brother, sister, business executive, nurse, university professor, etc., or he or she may be from a different culture than those of health professionals involved in his or her care. Considering those characteristics when working with the patient is an essential part of what it means to be a critical thinker. When recognizing this contextual component of the patient's situation, you are able to account for cultural differences, varied responses to his or her illnesses, his or her individualized behaviors, and any personal idiosyncrasies that can affect the nursing care.

A relevant question that you might ask is, how is critical thinking related to the preceptorship experience? Critical thinking or the development and promotion of critical thinking are integral to the success of the preceptorship experience. If you consider that the major goal of undergraduate education is to prepare graduates who have the ability to be able to think critically, then any approach used to teach students must be shaped to foster critical thinking. The preceptorship experience is the major approach to teaching nursing students in the practice setting. Subsequently, it must be assumed that preceptorship not only prepares preceptees to become competent nurses but also promotes and fosters their critical-thinking ability (Myrick, 2002).

As a preceptor, there are many things you can do to promote and foster the critical-thinking abilities of your preceptees. The climate you create for the preceptee to feel comfortable enough to be able to think critically is discussed. We also discuss your part in role modeling, guiding, facilitating, prioritizing, and questioning—all of which you can use daily to help promote critical thinking (see Appendix D).

The Climate You Create

As discussed, it is extremely important that you be attentive to the environment into which your preceptee has been thrust. Although for you it may be an environment in which you are comfortable, for the preceptees, the practice environment can be daunting, particularly if they have never worked there before. Therefore, it is important that you be aware of the effect that the unit has on the preceptees' abilities to function and think. The level of preceptees' anxieties is directly related to the kind of thinking that can occur. The more anxious your preceptees are, the less likely it is that they will be able to think. When you value, support, and genuinely work with your preceptees, as opposed to telling them what to do, you lay the foundation for a constructive learning climate that contributes to the promotion of critical thinking (Myrick, 2002; Myrick & Yonge, 2001).

Role Modeling

There are many other things that you can also do as preceptor to promote your preceptee's critical thinking. For example, in your behavior, you can role model critical thinking. However, as a role model, you cannot be viewed as threatening or intimidating by the preceptee (Brookfield, 1987).

You must be seen as accessible, supportive, and real. In a recent study examining the promotion of student critical thinking, one student said, "It's not like she's an authority over me...She treats me very equal to her, wanting to know my opinion about things" (Myrick, 1998, p. 80). When you conduct your everyday work in the practice setting, the preceptee watches how you deal with various patient situations. How you carry out your nursing care, work though patient situations, and arrive at particular decisions influences preceptees' behavior and thinking in similar circumstances. In other words, you become a role model for the kind of thinking and doing preceptees will subsequently imitate. Make no mistake—preceptees are constantly observing you. They will, in turn, strive to emulate the kind of thinking and behavior that you consistently display. As one preceptee stated, "I think I've got some knowledge myself just from watching what she does" (Myrick, 2002, p. 160). To be a good role model you must be clear in your communication, consistent in your behavior, open to different ways of thinking about situations, and specific in what you require from your preceptees. As one student said about her preceptor, "She really knows her stuff, and she gets it across" (Myrick, 1998, p. 81). By modeling critical thinking in your everyday actions, you "can do much to encourage this frame of mind in [your] students," (Meyers, 1986, p. 47).

Guiding

The individual guidance that you provide daily to your preceptees is a major factor in enabling them to think critically as they conduct their nursing care. In a recent study, one preceptee said, "I guess you'd call her [preceptor] a safety net because if you need help or you need a question answered you have someone right there" (Myrick, 2002, p. 160). When you tailor your preceptees' patient assignments to fit their individual learning needs, when you show them when and how to organize their nursing care, and when you optimize any available learning opportunities, you encourage your preceptees to develop their critical-thinking abilities. Your guidance in providing meaningful learning experiences, teaching, giving feedback, and validating psychomotor competencies (administration of injections, changing their patients' dressings, regulating the IV fluids intake, measuring urinary output, etc.) fosters the development of clinical judgment or preceptees' ability to assess patient situations and arrive at reasonable and appropriate decisions about the kind of action that is required. One preceptor stated, "They [preceptees] do need that resource [the preceptor]. They just couldn't survive. It's essential they have somebody with them" (Myrick, 1998, p. 93).

Facilitating

Although guiding and facilitating may seem to be the same, there is a subtle difference. In a recent study involving the preceptorship experience, guiding refers to showing someone the way to do something or advising him or her on the proper course of action. On the other hand, facilitating means to make a course of action or situation easy to achieve or to assist the preceptee to achieve individual goals and learning objectives. For example, as a preceptor, you facilitate preceptees when you draw on your own expertise and experience to pave the way for their experiences. In guiding preceptees, you provide meaningful learning experiences in teaching and validating psychomotor competencies, fostering the development of their clinical judgment, and giving immediate feedback to them on their performances (Myrick, 1998) (see Box 5-2).

Another way you can foster your preceptees' critical thinking is through facilitating as opposed to directing. To facilitate means you strive to make things easy for preceptees in their learning. In other words, you are not throwing obstacles in their way. Unlike the more traditional teaching approach, by facilitating your preceptees, you provide the freedom for them to develop in their competence and confidence and enable them to become more flexible and independent in their practice (Burrows, 1997). Through interaction with your preceptees, you can facilitate goal setting, with expectations within the preceptees' grasp; often it may be a case of agreeing on what goals are possible rather than what goals

---

B o x   5 - 2

Practical Information: Facilitating and Guiding

Facilitating

• Paves the way for preceptorship experiences
• Identifies learning needs with preceptee
• Defines specific goals to accomplish
• Evaluates achievement of goals and objectives

Guiding

• Shows the way to achieve success
• Tailors experiences for the preceptee to achieve learning objectives
• Optimizes learning opportunities in the practice setting

are ideal (Burnard, 1992). By facilitating preceptees, you are paving the way for them to grow and develop. You allow them the opportunity to discover what they need to achieve and what they need to know in their clinical practice. Such an approach serves to enable them to think critically when conducting their nursing care (Myrick, 2002).

Prioritizing

Prioritizing is another way you assist your preceptees in the development of their critical thinking. Organizational ability and priority setting are fundamental to professional practice. It is through these competencies that the nurse circumvents inefficient and potentially dangerous approaches to problem solving and clinical decision making. In other words, those activities that must be completed immediately are done so before those activities that can wait. As preceptor, one of the most common problems you will face, particularly with beginning preceptees, is their lack of ability to organize and complete their work in a timely fashion (Myrick, 2002). Preceptees frequently have difficulty defining what is important or what should be done first and why. At the beginning of their practice experiences, preceptees must learn to decide which activities require action, or what is normal and what is abnormal. In other words, they have not yet mastered the ability to think critically through the process of organizing their nursing care. You assist preceptees to develop that critical-thinking ability by prioritizing with them at the beginning of the shift, reviewing what is essential to do at the moment, discussing what must be completed on schedule and what must be accomplished during the shift, and exploring what would be nice to do but not essential to do (Morrow, 1984). This process allows them to sort through the countless activities that must be completed and allows them to establish a sense of order to their thinking and work.

Questioning

Finally, another effective way to help preceptees develop their critical-thinking abilities is through questioning. Questioning is fundamental to learning. It not only enables preceptees to elevate their level of thinking but also enables them to deal intelligently with their world (Hunkins, 1989). Your questions to preceptees can help to direct their thinking process, provoke interest, stimulate and challenge them, promote discussion, and evaluate their learning. The practice setting offers rich oppor-

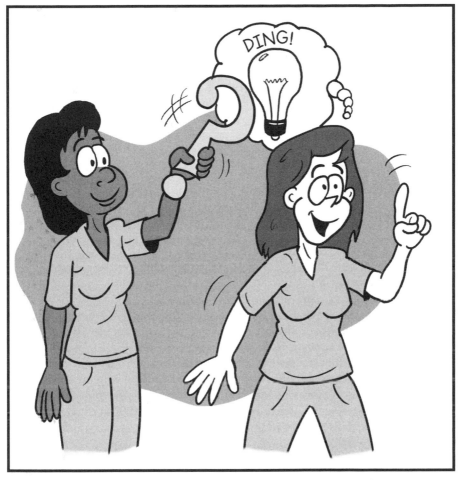

Your questions to preceptees can help direct their thinking process, provoke interest, stimulate, challenge, and promote discussion.

tunities for enabling critical thinking through the use of questions. You are in a prime position to challenge the way preceptees think by encouraging them to justify or clarify their explanations and decision making, helping them to resolve different dilemmas that they encounter, and facilitating them to develop originality of thought.

Although questioning is important, the kind of questions that you ask is also essential to promote critical thinking. In the preceptorship experience, skilled questioning has many positive implications (Myrick & Yonge, 2002). For example, when preceptees are skillfully questioned, they must demonstrate what they know regarding their knowledge base, discuss their individual perspectives, and reflect on critical issues that they may not have previously examined. When questioned, they must also apply theoretical knowledge to patient situations and provide the rationale underlying their understanding of the circumstances. As well, questioning affords preceptees the opportunity to correct or clarify any misconceptions. Your questioning can trigger preceptees to think critically and enhance their problem-solving and clinical decision-making abilities by stimulating the highest level of thought processing. Careful questioning and one-on-one discussions with your preceptees about patient care enable preceptees to think critically (Myrick & Yonge, 2002; Oermann, 1997). By questioning their actions, you not only spark their intellectual curiosity but also promote their recognition of inconsistencies in nursing care and their awareness of irregularities and differences between patient situations (Myrick & Yonge, 2002). Preceptees become enabled to deal confidently and competently with the daily complexities of nursing care. For example, in a recent study involving preceptorship and critical thinking, one preceptor described how she fostered her preceptee to think critically through her questioning: "If we have a cardiac patient, okay, what are the three main arteries, what is the problem, what can you anticipate? I want you to come back and tell me what medications will work for this or not. If we have a trauma, okay, what are your ABCs? Tell me about the airway, the lungs, what do you see? So she tells me, and I see how far her knowledge has come, and then I try and expand on it or we research it together" (Myrick, 2002, p. 161). Here's another example: "Okay when is it [patient's condition] acutely urgent? And she [preceptee] stopped and thought. Okay, now you're assuming you see a man arriving with back pain and you see that he's got renal colic. Well, we walked through the process, for example, when it's urgent it could be an aneurysm. You can assume. Stop and think about it. Don't assume that this patient has renal colic. He's grey, he's sweaty, and he's got a low blood pressure. Change your opinion. Now tell me what we could be working with" (Myrick, 2002, p. 161).

• Fostering Preceptee Autonomy

Your role in promoting the preceptee's autonomy or independence is pivotal. Although the preceptorship experience is required to be stimulating and disciplined, it should also be a "humanistic one which is authentic, supportive and caring" (Reilly & Oermann, 1992, p. 45). Only through this kind of experience can preceptees begin to develop a sense of competence and confidence in achieving autonomy as they conduct their nursing care.

Valuing Preceptees

An important factor in creating a humanistic approach is for you as preceptor to value the preceptees for their own selves. Moreover, accept them as intelligent individuals who bring with them their own unique life experiences and perspectives. Do not assume that because they are in a student role that they do not have anything to contribute (Brookfield, 1997). You can achieve this valuing by being approachable, open, and respectful of their individual perspectives. Despite that preceptees may be neophytes to the practice setting, they nevertheless must be recognized and valued as colleagues who are "equal human beings with ideas and opinions of their own" (Manley, 1997, p. 24). Valuing goes a long way in contributing to the preceptees' self-confidence and ultimate independence. In a research study, a preceptee said, "She's treated me like a colleague and not a student" (Myrick, 1998, p. 60). This statement reflects what many preceptees believe: that it means a great deal to be treated with respect and valued for their contribution when in the preceptee role. Preceptees are vulnerable. Their learning occurs in a most public forum. For example, preceptees must learn in front of you, other nurses, students, physicians, the patients to whom they are assigned and their families, other health care professionals, and numerous others. Therefore, they are extremely sensitive to any type of criticism and always cognizant of making a mistake, as reflected in one preceptee's words, "I've never felt I've had a stupid question with her [preceptor]" (Myrick, 2002, p. 159). Such a comment speaks volumes. As one preceptor so eloquently described, "I think they [preceptees] do worse if they feel intimidated and they're not allowed to make mistakes. If they're really uptight with you...they're not going to learn. All they're worried about is making mistakes, and they're just going to learn how to survive" (Myrick, 2002, p. 159). Making the preceptees feel valued allows them to thrive in the experience.

Collaboration

As alluded to, your approach to the preceptee is pivotal to his or her development as a practicing nurse and to the ultimate success of the preceptorship experience. Therefore, it is critical that you develop the ability to work collaboratively with the preceptee. Such an approach contributes to creating a safe environment, one in which preceptees feel that they truly are a part of the nursing team and not simply visitors or, worse still, outsiders. By being open and collaborative and communicating honestly with them, you create a sense of the preceptee's trust in you that can result in their true autonomy.

• Other Teaching-Learning Strategies

The preceptorship experience socializes the nursing student or novice nurse to the realities of the practice setting. It grooms the preceptee to assume the responsibilities of a professional nurse. However, preceptorship, as discussed, is also about teaching-learning. As we have seen, integral to that process are the various teaching strategies you draw on to promote critical thinking and the patient assignments you select daily. In addition, there are several strategies you have at your disposal that you may wish to use. One is the preclinical and postclinical conference. It is also referred to as a prediscussion and postdiscussion. The original preconference and postconferences generally involved a group of students. However, in the preceptorship experience, this is usually not the case because of the one-to-one assignment and corresponding relationship. Others strategies include, but are not limited to, self-directed learning activities, attendance at medical/nursing rounds, and impromptu observations (see Box 5-3).

Prediscussion and Postdiscussion Time

Traditionally, the preclinical and postclinical conference served as an important teaching resource in the practice setting. For decades, clinical instructors religiously scheduled these conferences with their students before and after each day of their clinical/community practice. This is an excellent resource for preceptors. However, rather than meeting with a group of preceptees, you usually meet with one preceptee. The purpose of the prediscussion is to give you and your preceptee the opportunity to connect one-on-one to discuss what is required for the patient assignments, discuss expectations—both yours and the preceptee's—for the day, and ensure that the learning objectives guide the assigned experiences. It is also an opportunity for you to ascertain how well the preceptee is

B o x   5 - 3

Practical Information: Teaching-Learning Strategies

Preclinical Conference/Discussion

- If possible, schedule for immediately before commencing shift.
- Review the expectations for the day.
- Address preceptees' questions/concerns.
- Clarify any areas regarding nursing care that are unclear.

Postclinical Conference/Discussion

- Schedule for immediately after shift.
- Review achievements of the day.
- Highlight the positive aspects of performance.
- Gently review areas of performance that require improvement.
- Respond to preceptees' questions and/or concerns.

With both strategies, be mindful of your approach. Be supportive, non-threatening, and encourage input from the preceptee.

Self-Directed Learning Activities

At times there will be little opportunity for more structured discussions owing to the nature of the unit, how busy you are, etc. In that instance, if you wish to capitalize on learning experiences for preceptees, you may wish to have them participate in a self-directed learning experience. For example, you may have them review the various policies of the unit and report back to you with their perspectives. Or you may assign them to conduct an in-depth review of a particular aspect of their patient's condition and present it to you and other members of the nursing team.

Attendance at Medical/Nursing Rounds/Observation Opportunities

An excellent learning opportunity for preceptees is their attendance at rounds. Arrange for your preceptees to attend rounds several times throughout their preceptorship experiences. It will afford them the opportunity to experience firsthand how the health care team interacts and addresses various patient care issues.

Observation opportunities are often impromptu. Although you assign preceptees to specific patients, there may be occasions when procedures are being carried out with other patients that might be of interest and would inform their ability as nurses. Have them avail of such opportunities, if appropriate.

adapting to and coping with the practice setting. On the other hand, the postdiscussion provides you with the opportunity to review the day to see exactly how well the objectives were achieved and how well the preceptee did regarding patient assignments, critical thinking, communication, psychomotor skills, etc. It is an opportunity to debrief about the day's events and to explore potential changes for the ensuing days. In the best of all possible worlds, the prediscussion and postdiscussion times should be "protected times" for you and your preceptee. This is quality time that is pivotal to the teaching-learning process. If such time is not made for discussion between you and your preceptee, then the question must be posed: How advantageous is the preceptorship experience to the preceptee's learning or your teaching?

Self-Directed Learning Activities

Another teaching-learning strategy that can be a benefit to both you and the preceptees involves self-directed learning activities. Such activities can augment preceptees' learning and experiences in the practice setting and concomitantly contribute significantly to the unit in general. "Self-directed learning activities are what the term suggests—activities directed by the students themselves" (Gaberson & Oermann, 1999, p. 108). These activities may be planned by preceptees to meet particular learning objectives or to fulfill individual needs. However, such activities must be designed so that they fit within the context of the preceptorship experience. It is often the case that you, the faculty member in charge of the student, and the preceptee get together to ascertain the feasibility of engaging in a self-directed learning activity and determine how best to accommodate such activity within the context of the preceptorship experience. Although there are numerous kinds of self-directed activities, probably the most relevant one to preceptorship is the independent study or special project. In either case, preceptees have the freedom to identify a particular area in which they believe they need further development and then proceed to configure their learning objectives, outcomes, and the evaluation process. Your input into such an activity is important. It is only through discussion with you that the preceptee can establish the appropriate parameters that must be established around the activity. Self-directed learning activities or special projects can vary from merely reviewing charts for the way in which nursing notes are consistently recorded to developing a manual for self-administered medications for patients and their families. However, the activity must be congruent with the preceptee's learning objectives and both of your expectations for the overall preceptorship experience.

Attendance at Inservices

Inservices, such as medical/nursing rounds, are an excellent resource for teaching-learning. They provide an opportunity for preceptees to learn the process used by the health team to discuss patients, their conditions, and circumstances. They also provide the preceptee with the opportunity to observe patients with specific diagnoses, review data related to their overall assessment, and discuss probable interventions. When there is an opportunity for your preceptee to attend inservices, it would be an excellent learning opportunity for which the preceptee will be most appreciative. Inservices can be either structured or unstructured. Often, the unit or the various departments in the hospital or community will schedule structured inservices. For example, there could be an inservice being conducted on the care of the patient with type 2 diabetes. Such an inservice would entail various members of the health care team, such as the nurse, physician, nutritionist, and patient, discussing various aspects of diabetic care. Preceptees' attendance would allow them the opportunity to engage in discussion and hear the different perspectives. The more unstructured inservice would involve something as simple as an impromptu discussion on the dos and don'ts of IV therapy and would likely emanate from a particular patient situation in which the preceptee is involved.

Preceptors often ask faculty if preceptees should attend inservices. If the preceptees are students, the faculty reason that they are in school all the time and need more clinical experiences. The ideal situation is to attend the inservice with the preceptee and then discuss with him or her what he or she has learned and how this knowledge will be helpful in his or her clinical practice. As professionals, the preceptees will be expected to continue with professional education, and attending an inservice is part of this socialization process.

Impromptu Observations

In addition to self-directed learning activities and attendance at inservices, there may be other opportunities either in your own unit or on other units that would augment your preceptee's learning. For example, if a preceptee would like to observe a procedure occurring outside the assigned unit, it would be entirely appropriate for you to arrange that. For example, when a preceptor determined that one of the patients in the adjacent unit was scheduled to have blood gases taken and knew that his preceptee expressed an interested in observing the procedure, he arranged for his preceptee to observe the procedure. In working with a preceptee on a cardiac step-down unit, another preceptor discovered that his preceptee was extremely interested in visiting the cardiovascular intensive care unit. The preceptor spoke with his colleagues in the unit, cleared it with the unit manager, and arranged for his preceptee to spend a day in the unit. In both cases, the preceptors took advantage of all possible learning opportunities for their preceptees so that they could maximize their practice experiences.

• Evaluation Techniques

One of the most difficult responsibilities that you will assume as preceptor in the teacher role is that of evaluator. As a preceptor, you are in a position where you are expected to judge how well or how poorly your preceptee is performing. The evaluation process is about balancing candor with sensitivity. It may be reassuring to know that even the most experienced educators find the evaluation process difficult at times, primarily because it involves making a judgment call on another human being. It is especially challenging when you are working with a vulnerable group, such as preceptees who are often given to self-doubt. However, the evaluation process can be tempered with the kind of relationship that you develop with your preceptee. If, as suggested, you create an environment in which the preceptee feels safe and trusts you, then the evaluation process becomes much more palatable for all involved.

To facilitate the evaluation process, there are several strategies on which you can draw to help you. These include direct observation, anecdotal recording, rating scales, verbal feedback, and preceptee self-evaluation.

Direct Observation

Direct observation is exactly as the term implies. It involves your immediate scrutiny of preceptees as they conduct their nursing care. It is what you do every day, and it is your most convenient and immediate source of evaluation. It allows you to directly observe preceptees as they adjust to the practice environment and see them interact with patients, families, staff, fellow students, and other health team members. You are in a prime position to directly assess preceptees' communication capacity and how well they problem solve, think critically, and execute their psychomotor skills. However, when you observe preceptees, remember that you are evaluating their performance according to the criteria specified by their learning objectives. By adhering to the criteria, both of you are clear about what exactly is being evaluated. In other words, the criteria create the parameters in which the evaluation is to be completed and serve to minimize any unfair expectations on either your part or the preceptee's part (see Appendix E).

Anecdotal Recording

To augment your direct observations, it is a good idea to develop the habit of writing down or recording your observations as you go along. These recordings do not have to be lengthy. It is prudent to write them down as close to the observation as possible. This helps you to avoid any inaccuracies. A good way to organize your recording is to first write down your observation of the preceptee's performance and then separately describe your interpretation of that observation (see Appendix F).

Rating Scales

A rating scale is designed primarily to provide a way for you to efficiently record your observations and judgments about preceptee performance in the practice setting. Rating scales are used most frequently to evaluate easily observed behaviors. They are self-explanatory and afford you the opportunity to evaluate different behaviors during a short period of time. Throughout the years, various rating scales have been developed to facilitate the evaluation process. Depending on the type, a rating scale can comprise numeric scores. For example, if one of the objectives of the learning experience is that the preceptee demonstrate aseptic technique when completing nursing care, then on a numeric rating scale, you may rate the preceptee as meeting this objective on a scale of 1 to 4. You may rate the preceptee as having completed this objective (1) unsatisfactorily, (2) satisfactorily, (3) above average, or (4) exceptionally. You will rate your preceptee in accordance with one of these numbers. However, recently many nursing programs have moved toward the use of rating scales that involve a pass-or-fail grading system, eliminating the necessity for the allocation of a numerical grade (Gaberson & Oermann, 1999). For example, with the same learning objective on a pass-or-fail rating scale, you would either rate the preceptee as a pass or fail. In other words, there are no in betweens, gradations, or degrees of performance. The preceptee either passes or fails the objective.

Although rating scales can be helpful in evaluating preceptee performance, you also need to remember some of the drawbacks involved (Gaberson & Oermann, 1999). First, always remember that the observation of and rating the quality of behavior are subjective processes, and preceptors vary widely in their judgments. That is why it is occasionally usual to hear one preceptor evaluate the same student differently from another student. However, it is the hope that the learning objective criteria provided by the faculty and preceptee can serve to create a consistent and more objective evaluation process. Second, remember that with time, behaviors can evolve. For example, at one point in the preceptorship experience, you may assess the preceptee to be unsatisfactory in a particular learning objective, whereas at a later point in the experience, you may discover that his or her performance is above average (see Appendix G).

Checklists

Checklists are a type of rating scale in which a series of steps are followed regarding the performance of procedures or completion of a particular intervention or technique (Gaberson & Oermann, 1999). Perhaps the most common checklists with which you may be familiar are those involving specific psychomotor or physical/health assessment skills. Usually, the behaviors to which the checklists refer are more specific than a rating scale. In the checklist, you will indicate whether the preceptee has completed the particular procedure or not completed it. When and if you use a checklist as part of your evaluation, it is appropriate to provide preceptees with immediate verbal feedback concerning their performance. This affords them the opportunity to review how they can best improve that particular aspect of their performance for their future practice (see Appendix H for a list of learning objectives that could be evaluated).

Verbal Feedback

Your verbal feedback to the preceptee is a pivotal aspect of the preceptorship experience. How you provide that feedback is also extremely important. Integral to your approach should be your projection of a supportive and constructive attitude. The evaluation process is a trying prospect at the best of times. It is good to remember that you essentially hold the fate of the preceptees' progress in your hands, and that is exactly how preceptees often feel about the process. They look to you to be empathetic to them in their preceptee role. As one preceptee stated, "I think she knows what it's like to be a student...I feel that she really supports me" (Myrick, 1998, p. 67). Whenever you provide feedback to your preceptees, it is important that you are sensitive to their individuality. As discussed, each preceptee brings to the role his or her background, experience, and perspective. It also helps if you focus on the preceptee's behavior rather than his or her personality. That way, the preceptee will not take your feedback personally. Always be constructive in your comments. It also helps if you discuss what the preceptee is doing well before engaging in a discussion about the areas of performance requiring improvement (see Appendix I).

Preceptee Self-Evaluation

An important facet of the evaluation process is the preceptee's self-evaluation, which is usually written. Usually, the preceptee expresses a certain level of unease with the self-evaluation process. The ability to evaluate oneself is a skill that develops with time, as preceptees acquire knowledge and experience in their practice (Gaberson & Oermann, 1999). As an experienced nurse, it is important that you guide preceptees through the self-evaluation process. You can do this by discussing their performance on an ongoing basis and exploring how they are meeting their learning objectives. Encourage preceptees to routinely verbalize their perception of their own performance. For example, get into the habit of asking the preceptee, "How do you think you did?" or "What are your thoughts on your performance today?" Such questions not only are engaging but also relay the message that you value their perception and in doing so you indicate that their opinion really matters within the context of the preceptorship experience. Because they are self-evaluating, it is also important to have preceptees explore the areas in which they need to improve. Having them identify and acknowledge areas for improvement puts the onus on them to take responsibility and accountability for their own learning. Finally, it is also useful to discuss the potential learning opportunities that the preceptees would like to embark on to strengthen their performance. Again, have preceptees identify specific areas and allow for ongoing discussion. This type of feedback and discussion again serve to confirm their role in their own learning (see Appendix J).

• Summary

In this chapter, you were given a snapshot of what it means to assume the teacher role within the context of the preceptorship experience. As we have seen, teaching is a complex phenomenon, one that is multidimensional. Although at times it can be demanding, for the most part, it is an eminently rewarding experience. Because you are an experienced practitioner, you bring an expertise and wisdom that can contribute greatly to the preceptees' socialization into the role of professional nurse. Through your guidance, facilitation, role modeling, prioritizing, and questioning, preceptees can develop their abilities to think critically and subsequently deal appropriately and effectively with complex patient situations. In this chapter, you were also given the kind of information that will facilitate you in the teaching-learning process. We have discussed the various strategies that will hopefully assist you in better tailoring the teaching-learning experience to the preceptees' learning needs. We also addressed the importance of remaining consistently connected with the faculty responsible for the preceptees. The evaluation process that is such a crucial aspect of the preceptees' development was also discussed, and sample evaluations were provided. The preceptorship experience is key to the education of nursing students. It is worthwhile remembering that in this role, you are preparing the future leaders of the nursing profession and, in turn, shaping its direction.

REFERENCES

Brookfield, S. D. (1987). *Developing critical thinkers: Challenging adults to explore alternative ways of thinking and acting.* San Francisco: Jossey-Bass.

Burnard, P. (1992). Facilitating learning, Part ii: The process of facilitation. *Nursing Times, 88*(6), 1, i, viii.

Burrows, D. E. (1997). Facilitation: A concept analysis. *Journal of Advanced Nursing, 25,* 396–404.

Facione, N. C., & Facione, P. A. (1996). Externalizing the critical thinking in knowledge development and clinical judgment. *Nursing Outlook, 44,* 129–136.

Gaberson, K. B., & Oermann, M. H. (1999). *Clinical teaching strategies in nursing.* New York: Springer.

Hunkins, F. P. (1989). *Teaching thinking through effective questioning.* Boston: Christopher-Gordon.

Manley, M. J. (1997). Adult learning concepts important to precepting (pp. 15–47). In J. P. Flynn (Ed.), *The role of the preceptor. A guide for nurse educators and clinicians.* New York: Springer.

Meyers, C. (1986). *Teaching students to think critically.* San Francisco: Jossey-Bass.

Morrow, K. L. (1984). *Preceptorships in nursing staff development.* Rockville, MD: Aspen.

Myrick, F. (1998). *Preceptorship and critical thinking in nursing education* [unpublished doctoral dissertation]. Edmonton, Alberta: University of Alberta.

Myrick, F. (2002). Preceptorship and critical thinking in nursing education. *Journal of Nursing Education, 41*, 154–164.

Myrick, F., & Yonge, O. (2001). Creating a climate for critical thinking in the preceptorship experience. *Nurse Education Today, 21*, 461–467.

Myrick, F., & Yonge, O. (2002). Preceptor questioning and student critical thinking. *Journal of Professional Nursing, 18*, 176–181.

Oermann, M. H. (1997). Evaluating critical thinking in clinical practice. *Nurse Educator, 22*, 25–28.

Palmer, P. J. (1998). *The courage to teach. Exploring the inner landscape of a teacher's life*. San Francisco: Jossey-Bass.

Reilly, D, & Oermann, M. (1992). *Clinical teaching in nursing education* (2nd ed.). New York: National League of Nursing.

The Preceptee as Learner

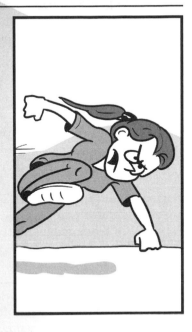

Learn as though you would never be able to master it;
Hold it as though you would be in fear of losing it.

Confucius

Even before you graduated from your academic or nursing school program, you were groomed to be a preceptor. At the least, you learned the principles of teaching and learning. You were expected to be a health teacher to your patients. Although you may not have been involved in a specific course on teaching and learning, you learned these concepts through role modeling, directed practice, and various classes, as well as through your own clinical experience. For example, consider the area of clinical experience and workload. How often have individuals returned to a health care facility for assistance because of a lack of teaching? To be more specific, think for a moment about the situation in which individuals return to a diabetic program because they have not been properly taught how to assess their glucose levels. Or think for another moment about the person who goes to the emergency department with congestive heart failure because of an excessive dietary sodium intake. To prevent their return to the health care facility, what they really require is teaching. Astute health care practitioners realize that effective teaching enhances the quality of life for patients and inevitably decreases their workloads.

These same principles of teaching and learning that you use for adult patient education also apply to your work as a preceptor. During the past decade, the literature indicates that on graduation, nursing students have been often ill prepared for the workplace setting. Subsequently, it has been suggested that those in nursing education must change their approach or teaching methods (Daigle, 2001). Therefore, the first principle to remember about teaching is that it is not about *telling*. Although admittedly there may be some telling involved when one teaches, generally telling is more about the teacher than it is about the learner. To teach means to think about the learner or to be learner centered. Some important points for you to remember about teaching include: (1) do not make the assumption that the way you learn is also the way others learn, (2) never assume that you know how others learn, and (3) if you ask others how they learn or what their style of learning is, with some reflection, usually they will be able to tell you. Therefore, this chapter focuses on preceptees as learners and addresses key ways in which you can engage them in the learning process. In particular, we discuss preceptees as active participants in their preceptorship or learning experience and how that participation can contribute to both their confidence and competence in the practice setting, thus paving the way for them to become confident and competent professional nurses on graduation. Because everyone does not learn the same way, you will need some working knowledge of the various learning styles that you may encounter with your preceptees. With this knowledge, you will be better equipped to engage your preceptees in the teaching-learning process by capitalizing on their own particular strengths or styles. Therefore, we provide you with some background or context as a foundation on which to guide you in working with the potentially disparate preceptee learning styles. We begin by discussing the different learning styles as described by various experts in the teaching-learning field.

• Learning Style

Just as you have a fashion or decorating style, you also have a particular learning style. According to Dunn and Dunn (1993), learning style is "a biological and developmental set of personal characteristics that make the identical instruction effective for some students and ineffective for others" (p. 5). Beauchamp, McConaghy, Parsons, and Sanford (1996) describe learning style as "cognitive, affective and physiological traits of learners" (p. 48) and note that learning style must be viewed within the context of the teaching-learning environment and that such a style remains constant with time. In other words, an individual does not learn in a particular way one day and another way the next. Pivotal to the teaching-learning process, therefore, is your ability to understand your own learning style, as well as your preceptees' learning styles (Garcia-Otero & Teddlie, 1992). If you are aware of your individual learning styles and you use that knowledge throughout your daily interactions, then your preceptees are likely to learn more, retain information for greater periods of time, experience less anxiety, enjoy the learning process, and effectively manage unexpected events. You will also experience greater confidence in your own teaching, knowing that the preceptee prefers to learn with a certain style and in a particular way.

There are numerous researchers in the area of learning styles. The two most frequently cited authorities are Dunn and Dunn (1993) and Kolb (1984). Kolb devised the Learning Styles Inventory (LSI), which is the most frequently cited tool in nursing literature (Haislett, Hughes, Atkinson, & Williams, 1993; Laschinger, 1992; Sherbinski, 1994). Essentially, Kolb (1984) describes his model in terms of a learning style cycle and the different environments in which that learning occurs. For example, one could start with a concrete, immediate, here-and-now experience, reflect on the experience, think about the experience (thus leading to abstract conceptualization), and then end with active experimentation or testing of the new ideas. This process is known as the cycle of learning. According to Brandt (1996), successful learners develop thinking skills that help them become aware of how they learn in terms of understanding themselves as learners, ways that affect the outcome of their learning, and how they adjust their learning when certain strategies do not work for them. The assumption is that everyone learns differently and at different rates based on their preferred learning style.

In 1971, Kolb advanced his theory of learning and combined the dimensions of the cycle of learning. For example, if individuals were concrete and active learners, then he called them *accommodators*; if they were concrete and reflective, they were *divergers*; if they were reflective and abstract, they were *assimilators*; and if they were abstract and active, he called them *convergers*. He theorized that nurses were most likely to be *divergers* or those who combined the concrete with reflective observation. Using Kolb's LSI, nursing researchers, such as Laschinger and MacMaster (1992), found that most nursing students have a concrete learning style. Other researchers have applied the LSI to nurses' abilities to carry out drug calculations (Bath & Blais, 1993) and have examined the influence of age on learning style and caution that not all learning styles when matched to the method of delivery necessarily improve learning (Cavanagh & Coffin, 1994). Convergers are more likely to embrace self-directed learning (Linares, 1999). Generally, because adults are naturally self-directed, four variables determine that self-directness: the level of technical skill, familiarity with the subject matter, a sense of personal competence as learners, and the learning environment (Merriam, 1996). Knowles (1988), a renowned scholar, describes adult learners within the context of four major assumptions: (1) they see themselves as self-directed and responsible, (2) they possess an accumulation of experience that is a potential resource for their own and for others' learning, (3) their readiness to learn is motivated primarily by that which they perceive as immediately applicable in their life situation, and (4) their interests focus on problem solving rather than on abstract content and theory (Holtzman, 1999). Of importance is a research study completed by Stutsky and Laschinger (1995), who examined the prelearning and postlearning style changes of students in a senior preceptorship experience. They concluded that there was an observable change in the learning styles of students that was attributed directly to the preceptorship experience, thus indicating that the senior practicum was a valuable and worthwhile learning opportunity. Ridley, Laschinger, & Goldenburg (1995) went even further to state that the preceptorship experience contributed significantly more to competency development than weekly clinical experiences during the year.

Dunn and Dunn (1993) developed yet another framework about learning styles. They described learning styles as comprising perceptual strengths and processing styles. Perceptual strengths, called learning modalities by Beauchamp et al. (1996), consist of visual, auditory, tactual, and kinesthetic strengths. Fleming and Mills (1992) in their study of learning styles included reading and writing as a category. If a person is a *visual learner*, for example, he or she prefers learning by observing and enjoys demonstrations, pictures, films, and videos. *Auditory learners*, on the other hand, prefer to listen, read aloud, and talk to themselves and learn best through the use of discussion groups. The *tactile learner*, a subset of the kinesthetic learner, learns by touching. A tactile learner will learn concepts best by tracing his or her fingers over symbols or patterns and by writing on surfaces with his or her fingers. For example, if tactile learners must remember a number sequence on their telephone, they will trace the positions of the numbers to facilitate recall. After a few weeks, if you asked them what the numbers were, they would have a difficult time recalling them, but if you allowed them to demonstrate the number positions, they would be accurate in their recall. Unlike the others, the *kinesthetic learner* learns best through physical movement. They have to do it to learn it. They will walk when studying, take notes, rewrite notes, and usually enjoy role playing (Beauchamp et al., 1996). Students learn more by doing than by watching others; thus, preceptors who engage students in discussion and hands-on learning rather than requiring them to observe will enhance their learning (Fernald, Staudenmaier, Tressler, Main, O'Brien-Gonzales, & Barley, 2001). In the literature, there are five approaches recommended to assist you in facilitating your preceptees' learning ability: strive to help them to learn, allow for their autonomy, introduce them to interesting or new patients, address their questions, and ask questions to push them to new learning heights (Fernald et al., 2001). Fleming and Mills (1992) also identified reading and writing strength as a style of learning by those individuals who learn best by reading the written material. These are people who will buy a new piece of equipment and will read the manual before attempting to assemble it. In the health care field, these are the individuals most likely to read the policy manual when they have free time.

You may well ask: Now that I am familiar with these different learning styles, how will I assess them in me or in my preceptee? A learning style assessment framework will assist you in answering this question. Following are three suggestions that can serve as such a framework to help you in your assessment (Griggs, Griggs, Dunn, & Ingham, 1994): (1) observe, (2) interview, and (3) formally assess. Observation begins with you. When you learn a new intervention or skill at work, how do you prefer to be taught? How do you spend your leisure time (watching movies, listening to a concert, or playing a sport)? When you have a problem with the computer, do you initially go to the help section or manual and read about the problem or do you experiment with various approaches? It may be useful for you to keep a learning journal and record for 1 week when and how you have learned something. Note, too, how you enjoyed learning the material. As a health professional, there is not a day that you do not learn something new, but how it is presented may not necessarily be tailored to your particular learning style.

Interview. Ask yourself questions about learning. Begin with your (or your preceptees') formal learning in grade school. How did you enjoy your first years in school? If you preferred recess to spelling, this will give you insight into your learning strengths and direct you to a kinesthetic style. Your choice of extracurricular activities and how you enjoyed them will also give you information. If there is another person who knows you well, ask him or her how he or she thinks you learn.

The last area is formal assessment. Unfortunately, you may not have ready access to learning styles assessment tools, such as the LSI (Kolb, 1984) or the Productivity Environmental Preference Survey (Dunn, Dunn, & Price, 1982). To assist you with accessing a formal assessment tool, a modified Fleming and Mills' (1992) tool, called "How Do I Learn Best?", is provided for your convenience (see Appendix K). Please note that each question is a parallel question. This means that there are 10 questions that ask you 10 times what your preferred method of learning may be. This tool has been used successfully in preceptor preparation classes. Before you try the tool, write down what you think your preferred learning strength is (*visual, auditory, reading and writing,* or *kinesthetic*) and then compare it to the results.

Other learning styles that you may encounter are termed *processing styles* and are divided into two groups: global and analytic. For example, global learners like to know the big picture. They want to know what they need to learn and why, whereas analytic learners prefer details and facts that are presented in an organized fashion (Morse, Oberer, Dobbins, & Mitchell 1998). Anderson (1998) linked the personality traits of extroversion or the outgoing person to the global learner and introverted person to the analytic learner. The most common processing style in learners is global. However, there are people who can alternate between styles.

• Personality Style

Another style that is worth considering when working with preceptees is the personality style. Personality style pertains to how you may be described as a person, for example, optimistic/pessimistic, introverted/ extroverted, or perfectionistic/chaotic. When coworkers describe having a personality conflict/clash with each other, such a conflict is usually based on the assumption that each is different in personality with preferences that are either not appreciated or tolerated by each other. For example, one coworker's optimistic approach may be perceived as flippant by a more pessimistic coworker. Therefore, the potential exists for a preceptor to experience a personality conflict/clash with an assigned preceptee. For example, if your preceptee is extroverted and you are introverted, or vice versa, it is conceivable that you could irritate one another. As preceptor, you assume responsibility for teaching preceptees and are in a more powerful role in the preceptorship relationship. Therefore, it is initially your responsibility to negotiate the differences in personality styles and to work with the preceptee to negotiate how the differences will be managed and/or resolved.

At this point, you may be wondering what your personality style really is. The most popular personality assessment tool used by professionals and nonprofessionals is the Myers-Briggs Type Indicator (MBTI). This tool is based on the psychologist Carl Jung's type theory and provides information about an individual's preference from four perspectives: *extroversion and introversion*; *sensing and intuitive*; *thinking and feeling*; and *judging and perceiving*. The scores on the MBTI can be used to determine decision-making skills, problem-solving abilities, group function, organizational preferences, breadth of interests, career suitability, and so forth (Hammer, 1990).

Various nurses have published the use of the MBTI related to departmental organization (Schoessler, Coneders, Bell, Marshall, & Gilson, 1993), interviewing skills (Heinrich, 1988), and decision-making styles for managers (Freund, 1988). Carroll (1992) noted that when preceptors were matched to novice nurses on the MBTI, an orientation program in critical care was enhanced and shortened. Biancuzzo (1994), who used the MBTI as part of a process involving the development of a competency-based orientation program, also supported this finding. The preceptors stated that the MBTI helped them "gain insights into themselves and their way of relating to orientees" (p. 101).

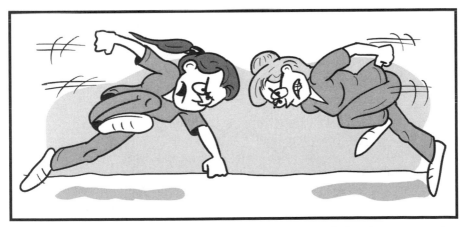

The potential exists for a preceptor to experience a personality clash with a preceptee. It is initially your responsibility to negotiate the differences in personality styles and to work with the preceptee to negotiate how the differences will be managed.

The MBTI can only be administered by psychologists or those who have had the proper training in the use of the tool. Comparable tools have been developed for public use but have not been researched for validity and reliability. As for learning styles, you can assess personality style through self-assessment, observation, and an informal tool. Box 6-1 contains a list of questions that you could ask yourself and your preceptee to assist you in determining your own and the preceptee's personality styles. You may wish to meet with the student before commencing the rotation to informally interview him or her.

Box 6-1

Practical Information: Assessment of Personality Style

These questions have been developed to assess personality styles. There is no right or wrong answer, and the questions are not related to intelligence. Rather, the questions have been developed to stimulate a discussion between you and the preceptee and to assist you in discussing personality styles. Please note: when discussing personality styles, focus the discussion on work-related scenarios. You do not want to force students to disclose information about their personal lives.
   When at work:

1. How would you describe your personality?
2. When other people describe your personality, what adjectives do they use?
3. Where do you get your energy (other people, solitary activities, music, etc.)?
4. How do you make decisions?
5. How do you solve problems?
6. When you work on a project with other people, what role do you typically take?
7. When deciding how you will complete a task, do you do it as soon as you possibly can or do you wait and see how it will unfold?
8. What activities do you enjoy doing at work?
9. How do you prefer to acquire information?
10. Would you describe yourself as a thinker or a feeler?

It is interesting to note also that research has been conducted to examine the relationship between learning and personality styles (Drummond & Stoddard, 1992).

• Preceptee as Active Participant

Now that you have been provided with some context concerning the different kinds of learning and personality styles that you may encounter, it is appropriate to look more closely at the preceptee's role as learner. With the knowledge that you have gained about these different styles, you can begin to engage your preceptees more effectively in becoming active participants in their own learning. Sometimes it is a natural assumption that the teacher teaches, or as discussed, *tells*, while the student, in this case the preceptee, becomes a passive recipient of what is being *told* to him or her. Nothing could be further from the truth. Learning is about being actively involved in what could be described as a discovery process. It is about being introduced to new ideas and different ways of doing things or about acquiring a new way of looking at an old idea. Learning is also about change. Once you acquire new knowledge about a particular phenomenon or situation, it inevitably changes the way you respond and the way you subsequently act. However, being an active participant requires a significant commitment on the part of both you as preceptor and the preceptee. An understanding of the different learning and personality styles provides you with the ability to tailor the preceptorship experience to the individual preceptee, because you can draw on that knowledge to help you develop a keener insight into how the preceptee best learns. For example, if your approach is not working well with your preceptees, you now know that there are alternative approaches from which you can draw that may better fit their learning and personality styles. It is this knowledge that will help you to create a more appropriate or learner-friendly environment in which your preceptees can become actively involved. Let us look at some specific examples.

You are working with Joan. She is a fourth-year nursing student who has been assigned to you for a 12-week final clinical practicum in tertiary care with a focus on the nursing care of adults after cardiovascular surgery. Joan is in her third week on the unit. During these 3 weeks, you have endeavored to provide her with patient assignments in keeping with her goals and objectives for this practicum that are both challenging and beneficial to her in her learning. During these 3 weeks you have established a specific routine. You meet daily with her to discuss her plan for the day and review her specific goals, objectives, and anticipated outcomes related to her nursing care. You also meet with her again at the end of the shift to address any questions or concerns that she may have related to the day and explore her perspective on how she can work more effectively during subsequent shifts. You are also available to her throughout the day as required.

During the first few weeks, you worked side-by-side with Joan to show her the ropes. Gradually, you brought her to a point where you believe that she should be able to manage her patient assignments relatively independently. You believe things are going well, until one day you are speaking with a colleague who says to you, "You know that student you are precepting, well she doesn't seem to be much of a team player. She never offers to pitch in. And she hardly opens her mouth." What do you do now? You are surprised at this outburst. Do you confront Joan and tell her to smarten up, or do you try to acquire more information to determine what is at the root of the perceived problem? In your interactions with Joan, you found her to be forthcoming, well prepared, and intelligent in the way in which she approaches her patient assignments. She is kind and caring to her patients, and her assessments are thorough. So what could this situation be about? In light of the knowledge you have gained concerning learning and personality styles, could it be related to one of those factors? When you review the situation, you realize that this could be the result of a personality clash between the colleague who had verbalized her concerns and Joan. Your colleague is what could be described as extremely extroverted. She is occasionally loud in her conversation and often quick in her responses. Also, she can be quite reactive in different situations. On the other hand, Joan is quiet and reserved. She is an extremely articulate individual and speaks only when required. With your knowledge of personality styles, you realize that it is probably not wise to have Joan work closely with this particular colleague. Therefore, you ensure that Joan works more closely with other colleagues who would be better suited to her particular style. You make the adjustment, and within several days, you observe that the situation has been resolved. Joan is fitting in well with the others. Although her demeanor is quiet, she continues to provide competent nursing care and works well with colleagues who complement her particular personality style.

Let us now look at another example. You have been assigned to a student named Tracy. She is in her third year, and this is her first time on your unit. Initially, when you meet with Tracy, you find that she is extremely talkative and somewhat flippant in her responses. You realize that Tracy is extremely anxious. You review with her what she has completed before coming to your unit. You take your time and review the kinds of patient assignments that would be considered appropriate for her in light of her previous experience. For example, Tracy has never had the occasion to catheterize a patient. In her previous rotations, the opportunity never arose. She thus expresses the desire to carry out this procedure while on your unit. Because your unit is a gynecologic unit, this will provide ample opportunities for such experiences. On her first day with you, you have assigned Tracy to Mrs. Johns, a 45-year-old woman who is in her second postoperative day after a total abdominal hysterectomy. She returned from the operating room with an indwelling catheter that the nurses removed the previous evening. Unfortunately, this morning Mrs. Johns is unable to void; she is requiring a catheterization. You inform Tracy that she will need to gather her equipment and prepare her thoughts, and then you and she will both proceed to Mrs. Johns' bedside. You meet Tracy in the clean utility room, where she has gathered her equipment. You ask her if she has any questions, to which she responds, "I don't think so." When you arrive at her bedside, it is clear that Mrs. Johns is uncomfortable. You proceed with Tracy to set up the tray and to conduct the procedure. After three attempts with three different catheters, Tracy is unable to complete the procedure. You subsequently take over the procedure and successfully catheterize Mrs. Johns. You then proceed to chart. Fifteen minutes later, you arrange to meet with Tracy for a debriefing session. You find her in the conference room in tears. She is in a high state of anxiety, saying that she feels terrible because of her incapability. You talk to Tracy gently and reassure her that every nursing student goes through this type of experience at some time in his or her program. Perhaps now would be a good time to review the event and try to ascertain how you could have done things differently. In your own mind, you wonder if perhaps there would have been a better way to prepare Tracy. Could it be that because of her particular learning style this was not the best approach for her? You have some time available right now, so you suggest to Tracy that you both grab a coffee and take the next 30 minutes or so to discuss how to approach such a situation in the future to maximize the experience for her. You begin the discussion by asking Tracy how she best learns. How does she study? What works for her on a regular basis? She responds by saying that she likes to watch people do things. She indicates that by watching, she comes to an understanding of what it is that is required and how best to go about doing something. You then proceed to ask her if it would have been better for her had she first observed you conduct the catheterization and then perhaps complete the procedure at another time. "Yes," Tracy responds. "I think now that I would not have been so nervous." Then, in reviewing the situation, you realize that Tracy learns best by first observing and then doing. Thus, the future assignments that require specific skills or procedures, if at all possible, can be arranged so that Tracy is first given the opportunity to observe before being required to complete it herself.

With both of these examples, the important point to remember is that you do have at your disposal the knowledge to assess the situation in terms of the preceptees' learning and personality styles. It does not take a lot of time, and once you have done this, it can prevent an inordinate amount of anxiety on the part of the preceptee and decrease your concerns as well.

• Encouraging the Preceptee to Engage in Dialogue

Another key element from the perspective of preceptee as learner is the preceptees' abilities to readily engage in dialogue. For you to help them develop this ability, it is critical that you understand their styles, as discussed, but it is also important that you create a climate in which they feel safe to engage in dialogue. The importance of the learning climate cannot be overestimated. The environment of the unit on which you work with your preceptees is a key element concerning how well the preceptees develop. If they believe that they are being treated like strangers, preceptees will shut down and basically work to get through the experience. As one preceptor described, "If they're [preceptees] really uptight with you and you're coming down hard on them, they're not going to learn. All they're worried about is making mistakes, and they're just going to learn how to survive" (Myrick & Yonge, 2001, p. 461). On the other hand, if the environment is nurturing, the preceptees will flourish. Throughout the years, numerous scholars have recognized the significance of how the learning environment contributes to the learner's ability to succeed (Brookfield, 1986, 1987; Flynn, 1997, Friere, 1990, Knowles, 1988; Mezirow, 1990; Myrick & Yonge, 2001; Yonge, Myrick, & Haase, 2002). It is also clear that the most effective environment for learning is one that is supportive, nonthreatening, open to different ways of thinking, and fosters a sense of trust (Manley, 1997; Myrick & Yonge, 2001). As the preceptor, you play a crucial role in ensuring that the environment is receptive to your preceptees so that they will feel safe enough and respected enough to actively engage in the learning process.

You also must encourage your preceptees to ask questions freely as they progress through the experience. It is through their questioning that you learn where they are regarding their thinking ability. It is through their questioning that you can also take the opportunity to respond to them and to challenge them in their critical thinking, problem solving, and clinical decision making. For example, when a preceptee asks you why it is necessary to change her patient's dressing three times a day, you might respond by asking, "Why would you think it is necessary?" Such a response from you will give you an opportunity to assess the preceptee's understanding of aseptic technique, wound care, and the effect that such a procedure has on his or her patient. It also gives your preceptee the opportunity to provide an informed perspective. When preceptees realize that they will be expected to ask questions, as well as respond to questions, they know that they must be prepared when they assume their patient care responsibilities.

• Preceptee Confidence and Competence

One of the major concerns when working with preceptees is that they become safe, competent practitioners. To achieve this goal, it is necessary that they develop a sense of confidence in the practice setting. All of the factors and issues that we have discussed, such as tailoring the experience to fit their particular learning and personality styles, creating a positive environment in which they can flourish, and encouraging them to freely ask questions, contribute to their development as confident and competent nurses. Your support and respect are also particularly important. Preceptees must feel that you are truly interested in them, not only as learners but also as human beings. They must believe that they are making a contribution to your unit. Your open acknowledgment and recognition of them will foster a sense of accomplishment and confidence on their part. One point to remember is that preceptees and students generally have a fear of failure. Thus, if they are not guided through the preceptorship experience positively and supportively, their fear can translate into a complete lack of self-confidence. One of the best ways that you can contribute to your preceptees' self-confidence and competence is by your example. How you conduct yourself with your colleagues and others relays a particular message to preceptees. The adage that actions speak louder than words is appropriate in this instance.

• Summary

The purpose of this chapter is to discuss more fully the role of the preceptee as learner and provide some context regarding the differences that you may encounter regarding learning and personality styles. Knowledge of these styles will assist you in working more effectively and efficiently with preceptees. The potential for tension between you and your preceptee can decrease greatly when you can recognize and respect one another's styles. By gaining understanding and insight into this knowledge, it is our hope that you will become better equipped in the use of different approaches that will assist you in facilitating preceptee learning. If one way is not working, then you know that you can draw on other possibilities. In addition to being aware of different preceptee learning and personality styles, you also must be cognizant of the learning environment. Your role in ensuring that it is supportive and positive will go a long way in encouraging your preceptees to become the active learners they must be to achieve success in the preceptorship experience.

REFERENCES

Anderson, J. (1998). Orientation with style: Matching teaching/learning style. *Journal for Nurses in Staff Development, 14,* 1–7.

Bath, J. B., & Blais, K. (1993). Learning style as a predictor of drug dosage calculation ability. *Nurse Educator, 18,* 33–36.

Beauchamp, L., McConaghy, G., Parsons, J., & Sanford, K. (1996). *Teaching from the outside in.* Edmonton, Alberta: Les Editions Duval Inc.

Biancuzzo, M. (1994). Staff nurse preceptors: A program they "own". *Clinical Nurse Specialist, 8,* 97–102.

Brandt, B. (1996). Cognitive learning theory and continuing health professions education. *The Journal of Continuing Education in the Health Professions, 16,* 197–202.

Brookfield, S. D. (1986). *Understanding and facilitating adult learning: A comprehensive analysis of principles and effective practices.* San Francisco: Jossey-Bass.

Brookfield, S. D. (1987). *Developing critical thinking. Challenging adults to explore alternative ways of thinking and acting.* San Francisco: Jossey-Bass.

Carroll, P. (1992). Using personality styles to enhance preceptor programs. *Dimensions of Critical Care Nursing, 11,* 114–119.

Cavanagh, S., & Coffin, D. (1994). Matching instructional preference and teaching styles: A review of the literature. *Nurse Education Today, 14,* 106–110.

Daigle, J. (2001). Preceptors in nursing education: Facilitating student learning. *Kansas Nurse, 76*(4), 3–4.

Drummond, R. J., & Stoddard, A. H. (1992). Learning style and personality type. *Perceptual & Motor Skills, 75,* 99–104.

Dunn, R., & Dunn, K. (1993). *Teaching secondary students through individual learning style.* Needham Heights, MA: Allyn and Bacon.

Dunn, R., Dunn, K., & Price, G. E. (1982). *Productivity environmental preference survey.* Lawrence, KS: Price Systems.

Fernald, D. H., Staudenmaier, A. C., Tressler, C. J., Main, D. S., O'Brien-Gonzales, A., & Barley, G. E. (2001). Student perspectives on primary care preceptorships: Enhancing the medical student preceptorship learning environment. *Teaching and Learning in Medicine, 13*, 13–20.

Fleming, N. D., & Mills, C. (1992). Not another inventory, rather a catalyst for reflections. *To Improve the Academy, 11*, 137–155.

Flynn, J. P. (1997). *The role of the preceptor. A guide for nurse educators.* New York: Springer.

Freund, C. M. (1988). Decision-making styles: Managerial application of the MBTI and Type Theory. *Journal of Nursing Administration, 18*, 5–11.

Friere, P. (1997). *Pedagogy of the oppressed* (rev. 20th ed.). New York: Continuum.

Garcia-Otero, M., & Teddlie, C. (1992). The effect of knowledge of learning styles on anxiety and clinical performance of nurse anesthesiology students. *ANNA Journal, 60,* 257–160.

Griggs, D., Griggs, S. A., Dunn, R., & Ingham, J. (1994). Accommodating nursing students' diverse learning styles. *Nurse Educator, 19*, 41–50.

Haislett, J., Hughes, R. B., Atkinson, G. J., & Williams, C. L. (1993). Success in baccalaureate nursing programs: A matter of accommodation? *Journal of Nursing Education, 32*, 64–70.

Hammer, A. L. (1990). *Introduction to type.* Palto Alto, CA: Consulting Psychologists Press Inc.

Heinrich, K. T. (1988) What's my type? Teaching interviewing skills. *Nurse Educator, 13,* 34–37.

Holtzman, G. (1999). The development of a self-directed module for orientation of nursing students to multiple inpatient clinical sites. *Journal of Nursing Education, 38*, 380–381.

Knowles, M. S. (1988). *The modern practice of adult education: From pedagogy to andragogy.* Chicago: Follett.

Kolb, D. A. (1984). *Experiential learning: Experience as the source of learning and development.* Englewood Cliffs, NJ: Prentice Hall.

Laschinger, H. K. (1992). Impact of nursing learning environment on adaptive competency development in baccalaureate students. *Journal of Professional Nursing, 8,* 105–114.

Laschinger, H. K. & MacMaster, E. (1992). Effect of pregraduate preceptorship experience on development of adaptive competencies of baccalaureate nursing students. *Journal of Nursing Education, 31,* 258–264.

Linares, A. (1999). Learning styles of students and faculty in selected health care professions. *Journal of Nursing Education, 38*, 407–414.

Manley, M. J. (1997). Adult learning concepts important to precepting (pp. 15–47). In J. P. Flynn (Ed.), *The role of the preceptor. A guide for nurse educators and clinicians.* New York: Springer.

Merriam, S. B. (1996). Updating our knowledge of adult learning. *The Journal of Continuing Education in the Health Professions, 16*, 136–143.

Mezirow, J. (1990). *Fostering critical reflection in adulthood: A guide to transformative and emancipatory learning.* San Francisco: Jossey-Bass.

Morse, J. S., Oberer, J., Dobbins, J., & Mitchell, D. (1998). Understanding learning styles: Implications for staff development educators. *Journal of Nursing Staff Development, 14*(1), 1–8.

Myrick, F., & Yonge, O. (2001). Creating a climate for critical thinking in the preceptorship experience. *Nurse Education Today, 21*, 461–467.

Ridley, J., Laschinger, H. K., & Goldenburg, D. (1995). The effect of a senior preceptorship on the adaptive competencies of community college nursing
students. *Journal of Advanced Nursing, 22*, 58–65.
Schoessler, M., Coneders, F., Bell, L. F., Marshall, D., & Gilson, M. (1993). Use of
the Myers-Briggs type indicator to develop a continuing education department. *Journal of Nursing Staff Development, 9*, 8–13.
Sherbinski, L. (1994). Learning styles of nurse anesthesia students related to
level in a master of science in nursing program. *ANNA Journal, 62*,
32–45.
Stutsky, B. J., & Laschinger, H. K. (1995). Changes in student learning styles
and adaptive learning competencies following a senior preceptorship program. *Journal of Advanced Nursing, 21*, 143–153.
Yonge, O., Myrick, F., & Haase, M. (2002). Student nurse stress in the preceptorship experience. *Nurse Educator, 27*(2), 84–88.

CHAPTER 7

Learning Opportunities

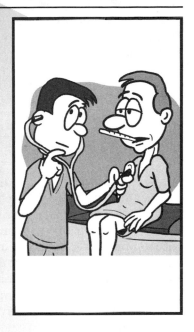

A wise man will make more opportunities than he finds.

Francis Bacon

As with any association or relationship, there are times when preceptorship is challenging. For example, there may be occasions when you will encounter conflicting situations among you and your preceptee, you and the faculty, the preceptee and the faculty, you and the staff, or the preceptee and staff. Whatever the circumstance, it is important that you resolve the situation quickly and constructively. Other times, your preceptee may not be performing competently. You also must resolve this situation efficiently. What about the student who is not progressing? What if the preceptee's behavior is ethically questionable? In this chapter, we provide you with suggestions concerning how best to resolve such occurrences to the satisfaction of everyone involved.

The situations discussed in this chapter are both "difficult" and "troublesome" and occasionally can be annoying and challenging. However, they are reflective of any situation in which people work together closely. Your approach can make the difference in whether such situations are effectively resolved. It is also an opportunity for you to learn to adopt best practices in dealing with any difficult situation or person. Therefore, we have taken this positive approach to such challenging situations and discuss them in relation to learning opportunities. What you learn from situations in the present will ultimately benefit you in dealing with future comparable complications and will equip you to do so.

• Conflicting Situations

The word *conflict* refers to discord or friction, and it is something that often cannot be avoided. Such situations can assume many guises. One that readily occurs is a personality conflict between you and your preceptee, an especially challenging situation because of the one-to-one nature of the preceptorship experience. What if you and your preceptee have different personality and working styles? Is such a situation resolvable or workable? Is the relationship salvageable, or should it be terminated immediately? For example, as a nurse, you are organized, meticulous, and motivated. You strive to conduct your nursing care in a timely manner. You have been assigned to work with a preceptee who is disorganized (as are most beginning preceptees), and who is also routinely forgetful and lacks motivation or enthusiasm. Also, from your perspective, the preceptee does not seem to be interested in connecting with the staff or the patients. Simply put, the preceptee does what is minimally required.

What do you do in this instance? Most important, you must address the behavior. It is essential that you address such behavior directly with the preceptee in question. As soon as you detect a behavior pattern, speak immediately with the preceptee about your observations. Be direct but gentle in your approach. State clearly what behaviors you have observed and how you have interpreted them. The key is for you to give the preceptee the opportunity to provide his or her perception of the behavior. You may be surprised to discover that the behavior is a manifestation of anxiety about the setting or is related to his or her lack of experience or fear of making a mistake. It may also be related to the preceptee feeling completely overwhelmed or even intimidated by you (see Box 7-1).

"One of the hardest things teachers have to learn is that the sincerity of their intentions does not guarantee the purity of their practice" (Brookfield, 1996, p. 1). In other words, as a teacher or preceptor, you may believe that your approach is fine, but that may not necessarily be the preceptee's belief. That is why it is important to take the time to talk

Box 7-1. Anecdotal Example of Preceptor-Preceptee
Conflict Resolution

One of the authors, while working with third-year nursing students in the
clinical setting, was surprised when she encountered what could be
described as a conflictual situation with a student with whom she had previously worked and with whom she had gotten along without any difficulty.
She found this particular student to be excellent in the classroom and laboratory settings. She was well prepared, conscientious, and personable.
Now in the practice setting, this same student consistently reported to
the unit unprepared to assume responsibility for her patient assignments.
When questioned by the instructor, she responded with vagaries. When
she was required to carry out particular procedures, she was disorganized
and awkward. This behavior went on for several days. Finally, the instructor
approached the student and asked her if there was a problem. The student's immediate response was, "You intimidate me." The instructor was
shocked. How could this be? After all, she was supportive and caring in her
approach to all of her students. She certainly did not perceive herself as
intimidating. The instructor immediately informed the nurse in charge that
she and the student would be stepping off the unit for about 90 minutes.
She then sat down with the student to explore more fully what exactly it
was that was intimidating her and how they could work together to
change things so that the student could feel more supported and less
intimidated. They also discussed candidly their individual perceptions of the
student's behavior and found that they each had a different interpretation
about what was occurring. Essentially, the instructor discovered that the
student was extremely stressed at the magnitude of having to care for
such sick patients and often experienced insomnia on the nights before
clinical, which subsequently reflected in her lack of preparation when she
arrived on the unit. In fact, the student was more fatigued than unprepared. The instructor and the student developed a plan that they agreed to
follow for the remainder of the experience. Throughout the next several
weeks, the instructor and student met regularly to discuss the work for
the day. There were times when the instructor believed it necessary to be
physically present when the student was completing certain procedures.
At other times, she believed that it was necessary to step back from the
student and allow her some space, but ensured that she was available if
the student required her assistance. During the next several weeks, the
student's behavior underwent a complete transformation. She developed
into the confident, well-prepared, conscientious, and personable student
reflective of her classroom days.

This particular instance was a revelation or epiphany to the instructor
and one that she has retained in memory to this day. It served to create a
level of awareness that she has subsequently brought to many other student situations

directly with your preceptees to ascertain the context of the behavior. Remember to be open, honest, and gentle when you discuss issues with them or when you must offer some constructive critique of their performance. When confronted with this type of situation, you remember the following key points: don't ignore the problem; address the concern directly with your preceptee as soon as possible; discuss your particular understandings of the situation and allow time for both perspectives to be voiced; once you have clarified the situation, jointly develop a plan outlining both of your expectations and establish time lines clearly delineating when you anticipate these changes to occur; ensure that you always take quality time to talk one-on-one with your preceptee; and to resolve issues constructively, "you must first be engaged with the [preceptee] in such a way that you both feel respected and heard" (Kottler, 1997, p. 36). No preceptee will be responsive to you if you approach the situation with an attitude of blame.

• Questionable Competence

Occasionally, a situation will arise in which you believe that the preceptee is not performing safely and competently. Despite the many discussions you have, the preceptee's performance does not improve. What do you do in such a predicament? Once again, your approach is critical. You must speak directly with the preceptee about your concerns and ascertain his or her perspective on why his or her performance is not up to the standard. The next step is to develop a learning contract. In the past, such contracts often were viewed negatively. Students who were performing unsatisfactorily were placed on what was termed *probation*, or a period of time in which they were afforded the opportunity to redeem themselves. The term *learning contract* implies a more positive approach to such occurrences. By entering into a learning contract, you are providing the preceptee with what is referred to as *due process,* or the opportunity to improve his or her performance before he or she receives a final evaluation and is graded on the experience. It is important that you apprise the faculty member who is responsible for the student and include him or her in the learning contract establishment. Learning contracts may also be used to organize the entire preceptorship experience. In the instance of dealing with a student who is not progressing as well as expected, it is an opportunity to assist him or her in getting up to speed.

A learning contract is "an explicit agreement between teacher and student that clarifies expectations of each participant in the teaching-learning process," (Gaberson & Oermann, 1999, p. 213), and it is usually in written form. It allows you to specify exactly what you require the preceptee to achieve to improve performance and clinical competence. For example, if the student is disorganized in planning and implementing nursing care, then it is essential that you discuss specifically what the preceptee must do to improve that aspect of the performance. Likewise, if you find that the preceptee has been supervised numerous times while administering medications and is still incapable of proceeding without supervision, then you must clarify with the preceptee what must be done to improve performance and complete the particular task without help. As with any situation, it is critical that you ascertain the preceptee's perspective concerning why there is no progress. Is it because the preceptee is incapable, or is it related to anxiety, fear, or some other issue? If the preceptee has made an error in administering a particular medication, it is a serious infraction of what constitutes safe care. It is incumbent on you to determine why the incident happened and how you and the preceptee can prevent future incidents from occurring. The learning contract can clarify for you, the preceptee, and the faculty clear regarding what types of steps the preceptee must take to ensure competence. Also important to the contract is the time frame. It is important that you agree on an interim time frame in which you will evaluate the preceptee on the aspect of performance that requires improvement. If no discernible improvement is evident after the time specified, then it may be necessary to assign an unsatisfactory grade to the preceptee. This process should be conducted in consultation with the faculty. The important point to remember when dealing with a preceptee whose competence is questionable is to keep the lines of communication open at all times, be clear about your expectations, provide time lines for improvement, and ensure that your preceptee feels supported in the process. The guiding principle for all involved is the safety of the patient—a factor that must supersede all other considerations.

Another area of concern that can arise is that of preceptor competence. What would you do if you were a faculty member assigned to a preceptorship course and you begin to question the competence of the preceptor assigned to one of your students? How do you contend with this situation? Preceptors cannot facilitate the teaching-learning process for preceptees if they are incompetent. For example, during your interactions with the preceptor and preceptee you begin to become uncomfortable with how the preceptor is guiding the preceptee throughout the preceptorship experience. You are cognizant of unsafe behaviors practiced by the preceptor. For example, you observe the preceptor change a dressing for a patient, with the preceptee present, and note that her aseptic technique is poor. Or, you are informed by the preceptee that the preceptor indicated to her that it was quite acceptable to administer a medication that she herself had not drawn up. The preceptee proceeds to describe an incident in which she had been requested to administer a medication that her preceptor had drawn up. In both of these incidents, it is essential that you speak directly with the preceptor to clarify the situation. If possible, arrange a meeting with all three of you to determine exactly what transpired. It is important that you approach the situation supportively and constructively. If there is a misunderstanding on the preceptee's part, then you are creating an opportunity to clarify things. On the other hand, if you find that the preceptor finds no problem with either situation, then it may be entirely prudent for you to remove the preceptee from that particular situation. It is also your responsibility to discuss the situation with the nurse manager, informing the preceptor of your intentions.

• The Preceptee Who Does Not Progress

What about those preceptees who are not moving forward in their experiences? Although they are not incompetent, they are stagnant. These are preceptees who can care only for the same level of patient each day. When you do assign them to a more complex patient, they flounder. They cannot cope with a more challenging assignment. Again, the secret to resolving this situation, as with the others, is to have open communication and dialogue directly with the preceptee. As we indicated earlier in this chapter, it is particularly important that the preceptees have a sense of safety and trust so that any constructive criticism that you direct toward them is not construed as a personal attack. As with preceptees who are incompetent, those who are not progressing will also benefit from a learning contract in which you delineate clear expectations and time lines regarding when these expectations are to be achieved. Time lines are particularly important in this case. If the preceptees are required to fulfill particular learning objectives, then it is critical that they achieve them within the specified time of the preceptorship experience. Always in these types of situations, it is prudent to involve the faculty member sooner rather than later in discussions regarding the preceptee's lack of progress. Often, faculty may have some suggestions concerning how best to accommodate the learning needs of preceptees so that they can begin to progress. However, even after this type of support, you find that the preceptee is just not progressing. In this instance, you may have no other alternative but to assign a failing grade to the preceptee.

• Unethical Behaviors

Of all of the challenging situations you may encounter, perhaps the most difficult will be those involving unethical practices or behaviors. One of the cornerstones of the nursing profession is that nursing care be carried out professionally and ethically. What happens when you discover that the preceptee with whom you are working has acted unethically—a most serious concern? As nurses, we are required to assume responsibility for the

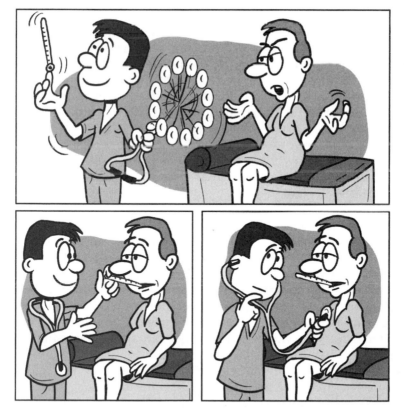

Preceptors should progress in their skill level during the course of the preceptorship. However, you may encounter a preceptee who just does not seem to move forward in the experience.

care of individuals and families who are frequently at their most vulnerable. Therefore, we are counted on to act in the best interest of those entrusted to our care. Ethically, nurses must demonstrate a respect for the dignity of human life and a respect for individuals, regardless of their cultural background, religion, or social status. What happens when your preceptee acts disrespectfully toward a particular patient? What would be the best action to take under those circumstances? First and foremost, it is critical that you address the behavior. Preceptees must abide by the same standards of practice and code of ethics that are required of all practicing nurses. As with the other situations in which you find the behavior of your assigned preceptee to be questionable, you must immediately address your concerns directly with the preceptees. Ascertain from the preceptees why they are behaving in such a manner and, more important, if they are aware that they are expected to act ethically and professionally at all times when in the practice setting. Once again, involve the faculty member who is assigned to the preceptorship experience as part of the discussion. The learning contract is an excellent way to deal with such a situation. Expectations can be clearly delineated and time lines can be established to allow the preceptee to correct the behavior, thus affording him or her due process. If the behavior continues, once again you may have no alternative but to terminate the experience and/or assign a failing grade to the preceptee (see Appendix L).

• Summary

Any situation that involves confrontation is at best challenging and at worst difficult. The key point to remember is consistency in your approach. Address your concerns directly with the preceptee or individual whose behavior is in question. Never, under any circumstances, ignore the behavior. Essential to the successful resolution of the situation is that you also seek the preceptee's perspective. It is always important to ascertain and compare your perspective with the preceptee's perspective. That way, you will develop a more accurate understanding and appreciation of what is the cause of the behavior. It is also important to involve all members of the preceptorship experience in dealing with the situation. The preceptor, preceptee, and the faculty must work together. It is particularly pertinent that you consult the faculty early in the process. One habit you must adopt in such a circumstance is documentation of your observations of the behavior in question, as well as your interpretation of the behavior. Written documentation is pivotal to a fair and equitable assessment of the situation. No situation is so difficult that it cannot be resolved. The key is to resolve any conflict to everyone's satisfaction, in this case, to the satisfaction of the preceptor, the preceptee, the faculty, and, ultimately, the patients.

Also remember that you have an excellent tool at your disposal to assist you in dealing with the types of situations discussed in this chapter. In particular, the learning contract is an excellent medium by which you can work together with preceptees to improve their performance. It is a written document that specifically outlines explicit performance expectations and timelines for the preceptees in which they are required to improve. The learning contract is a more positive approach for dealing with preceptees who experience difficulty in the preceptorship experience. It also is an excellent learning opportunity for all involved.

REFERENCES

Brookfield, S. D. (1996). *Becoming a critically reflective teacher*. San Francisco: Jossey-Bass.

Gaberson, K. B., & Oermann, M. H. (1999). *Clinical teaching strategies in nursing*. New York: Springer.

Kottler, J. A. (1997). *Success with challenging students. Practical skills for counselors*. Thousand Oaks, CA: Corwin Press, Inc.

CHAPTER 8

Communication

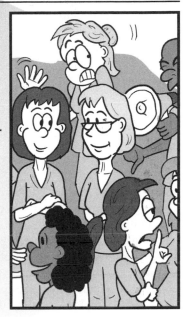

The limits of my language are the limits of my world.

Ludwig Wittgenstein

"Communication is defined as an imparting or conveying of knowledge or information from a source to a receiver" (Cantor, 1992, p. 17). It is a reciprocal sharing of ideas, opinions, information, and emotions. However, unless knowledge or information is presented and received, communication cannot and will not occur. Therefore, to be an effective preceptor, you must be able to express your ideas clearly and succinctly. It is only through effective communication that you and your preceptee can come to a working knowledge and understanding of one another. It is accurate to say that effective communication is the key to the success of the preceptorship relationship. Keeping the lines of communication open is key to how well the preceptorship experience evolves.

Because you are one of the principal players in the preceptorship experience, you must encourage your preceptee to communicate effectively, which is an essential requisite for safe, competent nursing care.

Although this might seem like a relatively easy undertaking, remember that frequently you may be working with beginning preceptees who are reticent about expressing their own perspectives or about asking questions and may require considerable coaching and coaxing from you. Therefore, how you communicate is an important part of your preceptor role, especially if you are to positively influence your preceptees' communication abilities.

• Types of Communication

Essentially, there are three kinds of communication. The first two are already familiar to you; they are verbal and nonverbal communication. The third is often referred to as paraverbal communication.

To be an effective verbal communicator, it is important that you keep your expressions simple and easy to understand, and, within the context of the practice setting, it is often a good idea to provide your preceptee with concrete examples when discussing various concepts and nursing care-related issues. This is particularly relevant to the inexperienced learner. The second type of communication is nonverbal. Interestingly, nonverbal communication comprises 55% to 65% of all communication (Cantor, 1992). The type of messages that you transmit through your gestures, facial expressions, and body language is critical. The worst thing you can do as a preceptor is to "suggest by a verbal response or some kind of body language (smirk, sigh, quizzically raised eyebrow)" (Brookfield, 1987, p. 72) that your preceptees' comments or questions are not valued. Such behavior can easily threaten your preceptees' confidence and easily render them silent, which will only impede progress and stifle confidence (Myrick, 1998; Myrick & Yonge, 2001). Preceptees then become reluctant to ask questions or voice their opinions, and they begin to focus only on avoiding situations that have the potential of evoking negative responses from you. In a recent study, one preceptee described it in this way: "You don't know what you can say and what you can't say. You don't know what's expected of you really. You have no clue what's going on. It's a stressful experience" (Myrick, 1998, p. 52). The third type of communication is referred to as paraverbal or "the way you make words sound—angry, happy, determined, sad, etc." (Cantor, 1992, p. 18). As you see, all three forms of communication are intertwined and are pivotal to your daily interactions with your preceptees. All three forms of communication are equally important in relaying your true value of and respect for the preceptee. It would not be an understatement to say that the way you communicate with your preceptees can make or break their learning experience.

• Feedback

A major facet of communication in the preceptorship experience is the feedback that you provide to the preceptee. Basically, there are two ways you can provide this feedback—verbal and written.

In the context of the preceptorship experience, feedback may be described as "the fuel that drives improved performance" (Parsloe & Wray, 2000, p. 123). Feedback given appropriately and sensitively can encourage the preceptees to become more motivated, increase their self-confidence, and develop their competence more readily. If, on the other hand, preceptees are continuously being corrected about their performance, they can become quickly demoralized, lose their self-confidence, and begin to question their own capabilities. Therefore, the purpose of the feedback is to provide opportunities for preceptees to develop an ongoing awareness not only about what they are doing but also about how they are doing it. In giving such feedback to your preceptees, there are two points to remember. First, always encourage your preceptees to provide their own particular perspectives on the situation being discussed. Then, follow their response with your perspective. This approach provides clarity and prevents any miscommunication between the two of you.

When you are working with preceptees, generally you are working with mature learners. As a preceptor, you must approach your assigned preceptees from the vantage that they are mature or adult learners (Knowles, 1980). Because they are adults, they will need opportunities to exercise some control or direction over their own learning, which is why it is so important for you to ascertain their individual perspective as often as possible throughout the preceptorship experience. That way, they will feel that they are providing input into their own learning, which affords them that sense of perceived control that is so important. As adult learners, their self-concept has a significant effect on the way they engage in various activities and how they interact with others in the practice setting (Farquharson, 1995). Closely associated with the notion of their self-concept is self-esteem, or the value that others place on the image that they have configured for themselves. That is why your approach to your preceptees is important. Because your preceptees are adult learners, they must be treated with respect and dignity and valued for their life experiences. They need acknowledgment for the competence that they derive from that experience. In other words, mature or adult learners expect to be treated as adults. To be treated otherwise would be detrimental to their professional and personal growth. If preceptees are treated with respect, they become more collaborative in the learning process and will be more quickly inclined toward independence.

As mature learners, preceptees also have their own particular learning agenda. Preceptees are individuals, and, although all are going through the same nursing or educational program, they come to that program and the preceptorship experience with different life skills and often with different goals for where and how they wish to proceed with their learning. "All too frequently one hears human service professionals complaining that a particular learner or group of learners lacks the motivation to learn about a particular topic. What this statement may more accurately reflect is a lack of fit between the teacher's motivation and that of the learner" (Farquharson, 1995, p. 53). In other words, take the time to become acquainted with your preceptees as individuals who arrive in the practice setting with a uniqueness for which you need to value them.

Verbal Feedback

In their daily learning, preceptees are required to carry out aspects of nursing care for which they may not have been previously responsible. Consequently, it is necessary for you to provide them with ongoing verbal feedback. For example, you may supervise your preceptee in changing a dressing for the first time or administering medications for the third time. In each instance, you will need to give the preceptees immediate feedback on their approach to the patients, their aseptic technique, or, in the case of medication administration, their appropriate use of the five rights. How you provide that verbal feedback is pivotal to how well they do in conducting their future responsibilities and nursing care. In other words, how you provide such feedback can make a difference in the preceptees' development of professional competence and confidence. The rule of thumb is that when giving verbal feedback to the preceptee, do so privately. In other words, it would not be appropriate for you to discuss the preceptee's performance in front of others. In particular, always provide the positive feedback first and then if you have identified areas that require improvement, discuss those after you have provided positive feedback. Never, under any circumstances, give your preceptee any kind of negative feedback in front of others. Take your preceptee aside, out of hearing distance from others, and discuss your feedback with him or her one-to-one. If that is not possible at the time of the particular experience that you need to discuss, then delay it until you have an opportunity to discuss the situation with him or her privately. An important point to remember is that no one likes to lose face in front of others. Giving negative feedback can be viewed as a form of reprimand, and, if given in front of others, it can become a source of great humiliation. Just as with any individual, dignity and respect for the preceptee should always be a consideration. If you remember to approach the preceptee the same way that you yourself would like to be approached under similar circumstances, you cannot go wrong.

Written Feedback

A second type of feedback that you will need to provide is written feedback. Unlike verbal feedback in which you discuss a situation immediately or shortly after it happens, written feedback reflects the documented observations and assessments that you garner on the preceptee's ongoing achievements or performance. As discussed in Chapter Five, there are many different sources of written feedback from which to draw, for example, anecdotal recording, rating scales, and checklists. However, as with verbal feedback, it is important to remember that when providing written feedback, first address the positive aspects of the preceptee's performance before discussing those areas that may require improvement. That way, you not only focus on those areas that may be perceived by the preceptee to be weaknesses in performance but also are first and foremost highlighting strengths. This approach is more empowering and affords the preceptee a sense of achievement and accomplishment. Such an approach is constructive and serves to create a sense of trust and safety on the preceptee's part. Preceptees realize that you are not merely concerned with their mistakes and know that although they may need to improve in certain areas, you are concerned primarily with promoting and encouraging them in the positive aspects of their performance.

• Communication Techniques

There are some simple communication techniques you can use to ensure that you listen to your preceptees. One is perception check. This technique involves observing a behavior, stating the behavior, and then checking with the preceptee to determine if what was observed was accurate. For example, a preceptor may watch a preceptee engage in patient teaching and note that the preceptee falters, because the teaching is interspersed with marked and uncomfortable silences. You may share your observations as follows: "I noticed that you were hesitant in speaking several times during your interaction with the patient and that there were marked periods of silence. Was it because you were feeling a little nervous about teaching that topic?" Another technique is paraphrasing. This involves stating in your own words what you heard or observed. If the preceptee states that he or she was uncomfortable, you might paraphrase by stating, "I noticed that you hesitated frequently, and I wondered if you were concerned that your knowledge of the topic made you anxious." It is important to remember that when you are giving feedback, you should be clear and direct and keep the feedback simple. As a rule, never give more than three points in a session. If more are given, the preceptee may become confused.

• Communication Challenges

In discussing the role of communication in the preceptorship experience, it is also important to specifically address the stumbling blocks or the challenges that can hinder effective communication. As a preceptor, it is important that you recognize these potential barriers and make every effort to avoid them and, if they do arise, to remove them as quickly as possible. Quite possibly, the greatest stumbling block to good communication is the intrinsic nature of the preceptorship relationship itself—the pairing of a neophyte or new learner (preceptee) with an experienced nurse (preceptor), both of whom are essentially complete strangers to one another. Add to this situation bringing both parties together in an environment that is often daunting, one in which you are required to conduct nursing care and make clinical decisions concerning individuals and families who are in various stages of crisis. As a neophyte in the practice setting, the preceptee often has little or no practice experience. Preceptees are also quite anxious and often intimidated by the health system environment. All of these factors can create considerable barriers to effective communication. As the experienced member of the relationship, your ability to identify these factors is essential for the creation of a conducive learning climate. Such a climate will, to the extent possible, alleviate or lessen the preceptees' anxiety and allow them to develop their competence and confidence as they conduct their nursing care. Only when their anxiety is lessened can the preceptees begin to feel comfortable enough and safe enough to begin to communicate effectively.

Interestingly though, your experience as a professional can also have a negative effect on effective communication in the preceptorship experience. Consider that you may have been away from the student role for several years. Subsequently, you may possess expectations of preceptees that may be beyond their capabilities and have expectations that may be unrealistic. As a result, tensions can arise between you and your preceptee. That is why it is so important for you to be diligent about immediately establishing clear lines of communication as the preceptorship experience commences and most important that you continue to ensure that openness continuously throughout the experience. Your ability to express clearly what you expect of the preceptee is critical. However, equally critical is your willingness to listen to and to hear what the preceptee expects of you particularly and the preceptorship experience generally. Effective communication between you and your preceptee is a significant facet to the success of the preceptorship experience.

• Preparing for Preceptorship

Preparing for preceptorship is similar to preparing for other kinds of experiences you may assume in your professional role. Some preceptors are approached by their nurse unit managers and asked if they wish to assume this role, whereas others are informed; this type of communication depends on the agency's cultural norms and prevailing management style. The management in your organization might have a rule that you can only be a preceptor once a year. If you are precepting a student, a faculty member will contact you. Depending on the location, the faculty member may also conduct a site visit. Usually he or she will provide you with a course outline, preceptorship manual, preceptor identification, letter of introduction from the student, picture of the student, and a letter of introduction and information from the faculty member. A preliminary meeting between you, the faculty member, and the preceptee is arranged so all of you can have an opportunity to discuss the preceptee's learning objectives, ascertain the kind of experiences to which the preceptee has been previously exposed, and determine directly what kinds of experiences should take priority for his or her learning over the course of the preceptorship experience.

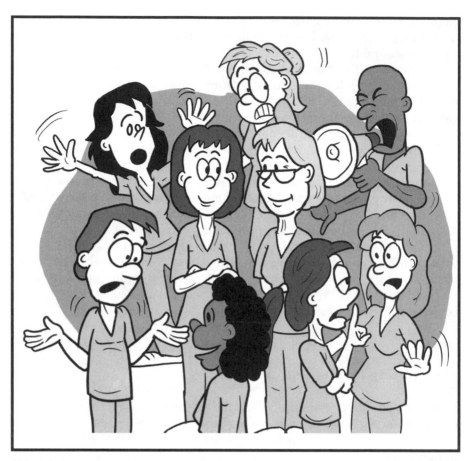

Although the nursing environment can be hectic, it is important for you to establish clear lines of communication with your preceptees immediately as the preceptor experience commences and that you continue that openness throughout the program.

A key factor in preparing for the experience is ensuring that the unit is also ready for preceptees. There can be nothing more detrimental to preceptees' experiences than to find that the staff on the unit to which they have been assigned is unreceptive to their presence. Although as preceptor you provide the primary support to preceptees, others in the setting also have an effect on the preceptorship experience. From the nurse unit manager to the staff nurse, from the physiotherapist to the physician, from the ward clerk to the housekeeper, all influence significantly the learning climate within the context of the practice setting (Myrick & Yonge, 2001).

In preparing for the preceptees' arrival on the unit, it is also prudent to ascertain exactly what kind of resources you will have at your disposal to facilitate their learning. Because staff members are a pivotal resource in the practice environment, your relationship with them is extremely important to the success of preceptees' learning experiences. How you get along with your colleagues can directly affect your assigned preceptee. In a recent study, one preceptee stated: "I think I lucked out. My preceptor is a good nurse. She's liked by the staff, and they know she's competent. I guess because the staff respect her and it actually amazingly rubs off on me. Because she's treated me like a colleague, it seems like the people she's friends with treat me like a colleague too" (Myrick & Yonge, 2001, p. 465).

The preparation for preceptorship is an integral component of the experience and is also reflective of effective communication. If the faculty member, preceptor, and preceptee do not take the time to communicate before the commencement of the preceptorship experience, it is conceivable that the experience could be unsuccessful. As discussed, it is extremely important that the three key players meet before the preceptee's entry into the practice setting. Such a connection provides the opportunity to open the initial lines of communication and to become acquainted with each other professionally. It also provides an important opportunity to clarify expectations. Allowing for such preparation is about good communication. Without it, problems can arise in the preceptorship experience, which could have otherwise been easily and readily prevented if the players had connected and communicated in this preparatory phase.

• Finding Closure for the Preceptorship Experience

Usually, at the termination of the preceptorship experience, you are required to meet with your preceptees to discuss their overall performance in the practice setting and to ascertain their perspective on the preceptorship experience. Therefore, it is important that you allow for quality time during which you can bring some closure to the preceptorship. Ideally, the final meeting will involve you, the preceptee, and the faculty member. At this meeting, provide the preceptee with feedback derived from your ongoing documentation. Encourage him or her to reflect on how the experience could be improved, what areas were redundant, and if there is anything that he or she would like to suggest changing about the experience for future preceptees. An evaluation form must be completed for the preceptee. Some forms include simple ratings (did or did not observe), and others are more complex and include numeric ratings and narratives. Regardless of the type of form you use, it is important that you know how to apply the form and understand fully the implications of your evaluation regarding the preceptee. Just as you do not like any surprises on a performance appraisal, neither does the preceptee. The most useful evaluation is formative, or the daily feedback that you give the preceptees on their performance. The term *formative* is an educational term that refers to the ongoing feedback that is regularly given to a learner to afford him or her the opportunity to make any improvements to his or her performance without the worry or anxiety of being graded. On the other hand, the *summative* evaluation is the evaluation that is completed at the termination of the preceptorship experience and does involve grading. It is in this final or summative evaluation that the preceptee is graded. This evaluation provides closure to the experience for you, the preceptee, and the educational agency. It also provides an opportunity to reflect on the preceptees' abilities to meet their personal objectives and the course objectives, to examine the process that they experienced throughout the preceptorship, and to say good-bye. If the relationship between the preceptee and preceptor has been a particularly close one, the preceptee may ask you to provide a reference in the future. It is not unusual at this time also for the preceptees to give a gift to the agency staff and to you as an indication of their appreciation for all your support and hard work. Preceptees give a lot of thought to the purchase of a gift and frequently consult with others about what would be appropriate. You may believe that a gift is not warranted. However, in most health care settings, gift-giving is part of the agency's culture, and preceptees truly value your contribution to their learning. After the preceptee has left the rotation, you should receive a formal acknowledgment from the educational institution.

Bringing closure to the preceptorship experience is also reflective of effective communication. When the preceptorship experience is complete, it is important that the preceptee, the preceptor, the staff, and also the faculty have a chance to say a proper good-bye to each other. It is a time for them to express their appreciation for the contributions made from both the practice and the educational perspectives. This is important communication. Without it, there is the risk of the perception being perpetrated that the experience is not valued by the educational institution or that the practice setting is ambivalent about supporting students, neither of which furthers the nursing profession's cause. It is only through good communication that such fallacies or misunderstandings can be circumvented.

• Summary

In this chapter, a key aspect of the preceptorship experience—communication—was discussed. How you communicate with your preceptee is particularly relevant to the preceptorship experience and can be the difference in whether the experience is a success or failure from both your perspective and the preceptee's perspective. Three different types of communication—verbal, nonverbal, and paraverbal —and how each contributes to a positive learning experience for both you and your preceptee were reviewed. When and how you give feedback to the preceptee and the effect of this process on self-concept, self-esteem, and overall professional development were reviewed. In this chapter, also addressed were some communication techniques that you can use in interacting with your preceptee. In particular, we described the technique of perception checks. This technique involves observing a behavior, stating the behavior, and then checking with the preceptee to determine if what was observed was accurate. Another technique that was described involved paraphrasing or stating in your own words to the preceptee what you heard or observed.

We also addressed the issue of challenges to communication. Invariably, when you have individuals, most often strangers to each other working together in what can be aptly termed a stressful environment, it is inevitable that miscommunication can occur. We discussed factors that relate to those challenges and made suggestions concerning how to best deal with these situations to the satisfaction of yourself and your preceptee.

The need for preparatory time before the preceptees arrive on the unit to allow you to ensure that the unit is preceptee friendly is a key factor in a successful preceptorship, as well as the need to terminate the preceptorship positively and collaboratively. Both preparatory time for and closure to the preceptorship experience require effective communication to translate into success for all involved in the process.

REFERENCES

Bastable, S. B. (1997). *Nurse as educator. Principles of teaching and learning.* London: Jones and Bartlett.

Brookfield, S. H. (1987). *Developing critical thinkers. Challenging adults to explore alternative ways of thinking and acting.* San Francisco: Jossey-Bass.

Cantor, J. A. (1992). *Delivering instruction to adult learners.* Toronto: Wall & Emerson.

Farquharson, A. (1995). *Teaching in practice. How professionals can work effectively with clients, patients and colleagues.* San Francisco: Jossey-Bass.

Knowles, M. (1980). *The modern practice of adult education. From pedagogy to andragogy* (rev. ed.). New York: The Adult Education Company.

Myrick, F. (1998). *Preceptorship and critical thinking in nursing education* [unpublished doctoral dissertation]. Edmonton: University of Alberta.

Myrick, F., & Yonge, O. (2001). Creating a climate for critical thinking in the preceptorship experience. *Nurse Education Today, 21,* 461–467.

Parsloe, E., & Wray, M. (2000). *Coaching and mentoring. Practical methods to improve learning.* London: Clays.

CHAPTER 9

Establishing a Preceptorship Program

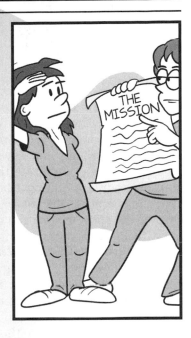

The only limit to our realization of tomorrow will be our doubts of today.

Franklin D. Roosevelt

As a preceptor, you are part of a preceptorship program. In other words, you are not simply teaching or being a role model to a preceptee on your own. All disciplines that focus on service to others include a practical or practice component that requires teaching and learning in the practice or clinical setting. Usually, this practical component is integrated into the curriculum, as is the case with nursing, education, social work, or medicine. In other fields, such as law, the practicum occurs after the student leaves the academic setting.

In nursing, there are many names for the term *preceptorship program*. Some simply have course names, whereas others are called internships (Beaulieu-O'Friel, 1993; Price, Dilorio, & Becker, 2000), electives (Brown, Hill, & Brouse, 1996), orientation programs (Brasler, 1993), or fellowships (MacMillan, Hops, & MacDonald, 1994). Some programs are unnamed. Lunday, Winer, and Batchelor (1999) describe how a clinical learning site was developed for undergraduate nursing students; a preceptorship program was initiated to provide a meaningful perioperative learning site for undergraduates.

Numerous different issues motivate the founders of preceptorship programs (see Box 9-1). Preceptorship programs continue to develop and have become a standard component of nursing education preparation and agency orientation.

This chapter focuses on the development of a preceptorship program. In describing that development, the authors use the metaphor of house building to illustrate the concepts. Before instituting a preceptorship program or building a house, you might ask yourself this question: "Why is one needed or warranted?" If the answer is because an area is chronically short of staff, the next question might be, "Is this agency having difficulties with recruiting to this specialty?" (Freiburger, 2001; Price et al., 2000). One strategy to address this shortage would be the development of a preceptorship program, with the assumption that a new staff member would be attracted to work in an area that would provide an extensive orientation and a preceptor who would be a guide, teacher, and safety net. As with house building, one of the initial questions would be, "Is there a commitment to the development of this project?" Although the

---

Box 9-1. Reasons for Implementing a Preceptorship Program

- To lessen job turnover by increasing job satisfaction (Macmillan, Hops, & MacDonald, 1994)
- To contribute to the knowledge development of students (Hunter, Dixon, & Lops, 1997; Lunday, Winer, & Batchelor, 1999)
- To decrease costs by increasing the quality of care (Beaulieu-O'Friel, 1993)
- To facilitate the transition from the student to the new graduate role (Gavin, Haas, Pendleton, Street, & Wormald, 1996; Konkel, Soares, & Russler, 1994)
- To improve upon the productivity of new staff (Biancuzzo, 1994)
- To develop and promote the confidence and skills of nursing students (Brown, Hill, & Brouse, 1996)
- To increase the recruitment and retention of nursing staff to a specialty area (Freiburger, 2001; Price, Diiorio, & Becker, 2000)

person in question may wish to develop a preceptorship program or build a house, there is a huge gap between the desire to achieve something and the realization of it. Inherently, building a house and developing a preceptorship program are endeavors that require a great deal of team effort that is directed by a clear vision or plan, considerable leadership, committed resources, and considerable time.

When people choose to build a house, they first determine several factors: where the house will be built, why they are building it, and who will build it. Experienced builders know that, first and foremost, they need to be committed to the project. If the builders are not committed, they may build a poorly constructed house with numerous structural flaws and other problems or they may not finish the house. Therefore, when conceiving a preceptorship program, it is not unlike designing a house. Those involved must be committed to seeing the experience to a successful completion. If that commitment is not in place, the preceptorship experience may be doomed to fail. The faculty, preceptor, and preceptee, as well as those peripheral to the experience, such as staff members, must all work together to create a climate that supports this teaching-learning endeavor. It is important to ask the question, "Will the preceptorship program have the required resources and receive the guaranteed commitment of the administration and those who are at the heart of the program?" If the program can draw from other established programs in the agency, it is like a builder drawing from the expertise of others. Resources from other programs can include preceptorship manuals, evaluation forms, or sample learning contracts.

When building a house, contractors have codes and specifications they must meet. Preceptorship programs have similar regulations. For example, they require nurses who are willing to be preceptors, preceptees who have learning needs, and a clinical or practice environment that is conducive to teaching and learning. Freiburger (2001) states that the preceptor is the major player in the effectiveness of a preceptorship program. However, one could argue that preceptorship program effectiveness depends on several variables. An agency may have preceptors, students, and learning opportunities, but if there is no willingness on the part of the nurses to engage in the teaching process, preceptees will be compromised in their learning and the program will flounder. In the nursing literature, authors usually are not afforded the opportunity to publish why or how their preceptorship programs have been less than successful. Although there is little discussion in the literature regarding why or how preceptorship programs have been less than successful, it can be assumed, like any other program, that preceptorship programs do not succeed because of inadequate assessments, poor planning, low commitment, lack of leadership in this particular area, or lack of funding and other resources (human, financial, and emotional).

Often, preceptorship programs are initiated and then intentionally terminated if the reason for their initiation is outmoded or no longer relevant, as in the case of recruitment for the provision of ample staffing. This situation also occurs when building a house. For example, a builder may wish to build a multilevel house and then decide that the costs are too prohibitive and then subsequently revise the building plan to make the house more economical. Therefore, for any type of program to be successful, it must possess the element of flexibility if the needs of those it serves are to be met successfully.

• Shaping a Successful Program

Regardless of the type, if you intend to create a program and invest a great deal of energy in maintaining it, you will want it to be as successful and effective as possible. Therefore, there are several specific steps that help ensure its achievement. The mission or purpose of the program must be explicit, known, and accepted by all participants. This step is known as the beginning or the buy-in phase of the program. A person in the agency may have worked in another agency where he or she had participated in or been aware of a preceptorship program or may have read about it in the nursing literature. When that person communicates the experience to others and demonstrates how the current agency would benefit from such a program, an educative leadership process begins.

When building, all those who would like to live in the house should have an idea or some understanding of the proposed structure or foundation. With this knowledge and insight, they can make recommendations to improve the plan and contribute to the shaping of the house.

The program must be described narratively. In other words, it must be clearly written so that anyone who wishes to understand it can do so without difficulty. This description or narrative serves the same purpose that a builder's blueprint of a house serves in that at a glance, one is able to capture its essence. This may seem like common sense, but for a program to exist, it must be documented. Through the process of documentation, the founders of the program then begin to comprehend each other's ideas and form a common understanding. A builder of a house would never start building without a written blueprint. The process must be clearly understood by not only those involved but also by those who are not directly involved but may wish to make inquiries about the pro-

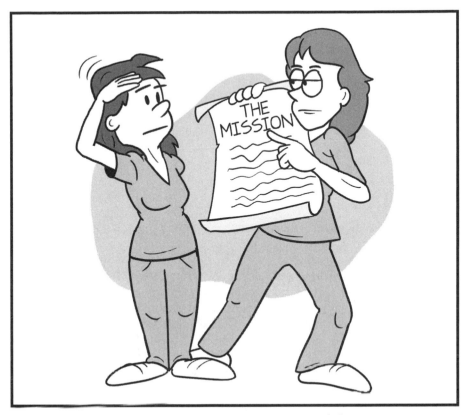

Safe, ethical, competent practice is the mission of all nurses.

gram. Programs may exist conceptually or in the minds of those who may wish to spearhead them at their agency but have not yet translated their ideas into a presentation to agency personnel.

There must be goals, objectives, and identified skills or competencies that are integral to the program. Agency personnel want to know why they are investing time, what is expected of them, what are the advantages and disadvantages, and how the program will affect their workloads. Furthermore, evaluation mechanisms are directly linked to the program's goals and objectives. How, when, and where the program is evaluated depends on the goals. If a builder is constructing an energy-efficient solar-heated home, the goal would be to create mechanisms and structures that will reduce heating costs. Thus, the evaluation or outcome would reflect a decreased heating bill. Similar to how a builder constructs such a home with a particular outcome, so too must those involved shape the preceptorship program. For example, if it is the goal of a preceptorship program to socialize nursing students into the professional role of the nurse, then at the termination of the program, students must reflect that level of professionalism. Or if it is the intent of a preceptorship program to orient staff nurses to a particular agency area, then the outcome would be that the nurse would reflect the required level of competence when evaluated at the termination of the program.

• Maintaining the Structure

Usually with time and with considerable effort, programs evolve successfully. The initial structure in which the program began may no longer remain. Therefore, programs must reflect elasticity, flexibility, and adaptability. Needs, personnel, and resources change. If a learning environment or structure becomes hostile, then it is more prudent to terminate a program. A new employee or student cannot learn in an environment in which he or she does not feel safe. Houses too are renovated. Some are made more attractive. Some are renovated to meet the changing needs of a family. If the house environment becomes dangerous, such as containing a natural gas leak, the occupants must leave the house until the problem is resolved.

Internal and external members must consistently support the preceptorship program. Internally, preceptorship is part of the entire agency, from professionals and support staff to patients. Faculty, visitors, and other agencies play an external role; although they may not be directly involved in the preceptorship experience, they may occasionally take part in or affect various aspects of the preceptees' learning experiences. Teaching and learning do not occur in a vacuum. They are part and parcel of a highly interactive and dynamic environment. One of the most concrete methods of supporting a program is by acknowledging preceptors. This acknowledgment may include hosting appreciation receptions, giving gifts, recognizing the preceptors' work on performance appraisals, or endorsements, such as a preceptor pin or pen. Preceptorship programs affect recruitment, professional organizations, teaching institutions, unions, and so forth.

The construction of a house involves many different players at various stages (eg, the designer, the main builder, and numerous other contractors, such as the electrician, the plumber, and the tile layer). The same is true in the preceptorship program, where there are numerous participants. Although the preceptor and preceptee are the primary players, the faculty, nurse manager, staff, and other members of the health team all affect in some way at various times the preceptees' learning. Similar to the construction of a house, different players contribute in some way to shaping the preceptorship experience.

Organizers of preceptorship programs must commence with the expectation that this program will be the best that they are capable of designing and implementing. Biancuzzo (1994) describes a program owned and managed by preceptors. This program is unique because change theory was used to develop a competency-based orientation program (CBO). What is particularly significant about the process is that a new program is the responsibility of those directly involved and not the responsibility of an external agency. In other words, the program that was a form of change was not imposed or dictated by others. Instead, those for whom it would have the greatest impact guided it. Because of their direct involvement and management of the program, they were an integral part of the process, effecting a culture in which change could occur without being threatening or intimidating. In other words, change was allowed to occur naturally. Such an approach is key in keeping with principles of change theory emphasizing that "the best way to manage change is to allow for it to happen."

Once a house is completed, it must then be maintained and sometimes renovated. This is also true for all programs. There are leaders or founders of preceptorship programs who initiate the program and then move on to initiate other programs. Their skill revolves around the initiation phase. However, ultimately someone participating in the program must take responsibility for maintaining the program. In the CBO program, the personnel who initiated the program are also maintaining it. Ideally, this should be the case for all programs. The task of maintenance invariably falls to administrators. How well they maintain a program depends on their priorities and workload. Such maintenance is conducted through observation, support, and evaluation.

However, preceptorship programs differ from other educational programs, such as teaching a specific skill. Preceptorship programs may be likened to a micro-nursing education program. All the structures of a nursing education program—the curriculum, principles of teaching and learning, and resource allocation—apply to preceptorship. However, in the preceptorship program, there are challenges in the area of consistency because preceptors may change agencies or assume the preceptor role only occasionally. Preceptee expectations, preceptor variation, and preparation of preceptors and preceptees for the program are also highly variable. Preceptorship programs are usually easy to initiate because preceptors are willing to teach and preceptees want to be taught. Unfortunately, that does not ensure a successful preceptorship program. In other words, although the willingness to teach may be there for the preceptor and there may be preceptees who need to be taught, there are many other variables that contribute to a successful preceptorship experience. Such variables include the orientation process, its availability, the availability of the preceptors, and the support and willingness of the agency to free the time to attend such sessions. On a more interpersonal level, how well the evaluation process is conducted is also immensely important. As discussed in previous chapters, evaluation at the best of times is a difficult process for both the preceptor and the preceptee. Compounding the preceptorship experience is the pairing of an experienced practitioner and a neophyte or novice nurse, and there is always the potential for conflict. How well such situations are managed and resolved are extremely important considerations as well. The preceptorship experience is thus dependent on numerous factors, all of which must be carefully weighed when planning and implementing the program.

• Summary

These are key elements that need consideration when initiating a preceptorship program, particularly if it is to be successful. There must be careful preplanning on the part of all stakeholders who must be committed to the program, from administrators to managers to preceptors, as well as the other staff. The mission, purpose, goals, and outcomes of the program must be clearly documented. The program must be flexible, dynamic, and housed in a positive learning environment. The program should undergo routine or ongoing assessment and renewal, a key consideration. It is not unusual to assume that once the program is initiated it will run itself. It is also wise to remember that a preceptorship program is likely to encounter more challenges than other educational programs because of the variability of the involved players. Lack of consistent preceptors can often strain the experience.

The preceptorship experience is a metaphor for all teaching and learning experiences, but with an added dimension. The preceptor requires all the competencies required of teachers in other settings, such as the classroom, while maintaining the ability to function as a professional in a highly dynamic clinical or community environment. The preceptee too must be a student of the clinical area and profession. To ensure that the preceptorship experience is successful, there is an onus on the preceptor, other staff members in the agency, educators, and administrators to create a positive learning environment. This is accomplished through the development of viable preceptorship programs, development of goals and objectives, systematic preparation of the preceptor and preceptee for the experience, and continuous support particularly for the preceptor and preceptee. Communication in all forms is key to the success of the experience: preceptees must be clear about their learning objectives and preceptors must give feedback, use communication strategies, and complete evaluations. Faculty members must prepare preceptors and students for the experience and maintain regular contact with them. Administrators must acknowledge and support preceptors during the preceptorship experience. Preceptors, preceptees, faculty, other professionals in the clinical area, and administrators have clearly identifiable roles. All must take responsibility for the experience, from role modeling professional behaviors to promoting critical thinking. A successful preceptorship experience does not just happen, it involves a complex number of activities as identified and described in this book. The end result of a structured, successful, and positive preceptorship experience is a stronger profession.

REFERENCES

Beaulieu-O'Friel, J. A. (1993). The nurse internship experience: A dynamic learning environment for the novice. *Journal of Nursing Staff Development, 9,* 24–27.

Biancuzzo, M. (1994). Staff nurse preceptors: A program they "own." *Clinical Nurse Specialist, 8,* 97–102.

Brasler, M. E. (1993). Predictors of clinical performance of new graduate nurses participating in preceptor orientation programs. *The Journal of Continuing Education in Nursing, 24,* 158–165.

Brown, B., Hill, B. J., & Brouse, S. H. (1996). A perioperative elective for college credit. *AORN Journal, 63,* 590–598.

Freiburger, O. A. (2001). A tribute to clinical preceptors: Developing a preceptor program for nursing students. *Journal for Nurses in Staff Development, 17,* 320–327.

Gavin, M. J., Haas, L. J., Pendleton, P. B., Street, J. W., & Wormald, A. (1996). Orienting a new graduate nurse to home healthcare. *Home Healthcare Nurse, 14,* 381–387.

Hunter, L. P., Dixon, L. R., & Lops, V. R. (1997). The University of California, San Diego Nurse-Midwifery Bridge Program: An opportunity to learn intrapartum nursing skills. *Journal of Nurse-Midwifery, 42,* 427–433.

Konkel, J., Soares, P., & Russler, M. (1994). A collaborative framework for baccalaureate clinical preceptorships. *Journal of Nursing Staff Development, 10,* 94–98.

Lunday, K. K., Winer, W. K., & Batchelor, A. (1999). Developing clinical learning sites for undergraduate nursing students. *AORN Journal, 70,* 64–66, 69–71.

MacMillan, K., Hops, S., & MacDonald, J. (1994). The nursing fellowship program. *The Canadian Nurse,* April, 31–34.

Price, M. E., DiIorio, C., & Becker, J. K. (2000). The neuroscience nurse internship program: The description. *Journal of Neuroscience Nursing, 32,* 318–323.

Frequently Asked Questions

When assuming any new role, there are always questions that arise. The role of preceptor is no different. Such questions can relate to any aspect of the preceptorship experience. While you may be reluctant to ask questions because you think that you should already know the answers, it is worthwhile to ask them anyway, both for your sake and for the sake of your students or preceptees. Some of the most frequently asked questions include the following:

What exactly does being a preceptor mean?

This is an important question. In a nutshell, being a preceptor means that you act as a resource person who is immediately available on a one-to-one basis to a nursing student or a new nurse in the practice setting.

What would I be responsible for?

As a preceptor you are responsible for being there in the practice setting and where appropriate to act as a *role model, teacher, facili-*

tator, guide, evaluator, and *guardian* of the individual student or nurse who is a neophyte or new to the practice arena.

What preparation do I need to be a preceptor?

If the nursing students you are working with are being baccalaureate prepared, it would be ideal if you were either baccalaureate or master's prepared. Because this is not always possible, it is most often diploma-prepared nurses who have considerable expertise and experience in the area in which the preceptorship is taking place who assume the role of preceptor. When preceptoring a new nurse to a unit, the preceptor is usually a registered nurse who knows the unit and has developed considerable expertise and experience in caring for patients in that particular area.

What kind of support will I have?

Being a preceptor usually requires the support from the administration of the agency in which you are working as a registered nurse. It also requires the support of your nurse unit manager or supervisor. In addition to this agency support it is critical that you have the support of faculty from the program or course in which the preceptorship is planned and in which the student is enrolled. You can turn to the faculty when you have specific questions about required learning experiences that are appropriate for the students, concerns regarding the performance of your assigned preceptees, and any questions that generally impact the overall preceptorship or learning experience.

Am I responsible for student evaluations? How do I evaluate? What do I evaluate?

Because you will be working with particular students for a designated period of time, you will be required to provide feedback concerning their clinical performance in terms of how competent they are. For that reason you will need to document the various aspects of their performance as you observe them over that period of time. As previously discussed, there are various tools that are available to assist you with this endeavor; these include anecdotal recording, rating scales, checklists, etc. Also, an important part of this function is to communicate on a regular basis with your preceptee and to stay in contact with the faculty involved in the course in which the preceptorship is occurring.

What do I do if I have a student who I think is not up to par?

One of the most important aspects of the preceptorship experience is open communication. It is through open communication that any concerns, issues, or problems can be dealt with directly, efficiently, and effectively. It is, therefore, critical throughout the experience that you meet regularly one-on-one with your students so that you can address how they are doing on an ongoing basis. Then, when it comes time for the more formal evaluation at the termination of the preceptorship, there are no surprises. In the event you do find that a student is not performing adequately, you need to address it directly and privately with that student. Never under any circumstances discuss a performance issue with a student in front of others. During your interaction with the student, it is important that you discuss ways in which he or she can improve his or her performance. It is important also that you designate a specific time frame during which he or she will be expected to improve performance. Finally, be specific about what will happen if he or she does not demonstrate improvement once that time has elapsed. Usually it will mean that he or she will fail the experience. Above all keep the faculty apprised of the situation from the very beginning. In fact, it is essential that you involve the faculty immediately because they can be an excellent resource and source of support when it comes to dealing with this kind of situation.

Am I responsible for giving students a mark?

While you will be expected to provide feedback on student performance, you will not be responsible for grading students or giving them marks. Grading is the responsibility of the faculty.

What if the faculty is not being supportive enough?

If you find that there is less faculty contact than you would like, it would be entirely appropriate for you to contact the faculty member directly yourself through phone messages or e-mail, or to have the student indicate to the faculty that you would like to connect. If none of these approaches is successful then it is wise for you to ascertain who is responsible for coordinating the course and to contact that particular person directly. Usually in courses that involve preceptorship there are sometimes up to 200 students who are assigned to various individual faculty. These faculty members are thus responsible for approximately 20 students and 20 preceptors at one time, and one of these faculty members would be responsible for being in contact with you. If no contact is being made you could connect with the coordinator who oversees the entire course to express your concerns.

How is being a preceptor different from being a "buddy" or a "mentor"?

While we hear the term preceptor quite frequently these days sometimes people may mistake the term preceptor with such terms as "buddy" or "mentor." During the 1970s and the 1980s it was not uncommon for students or nurses to be "buddied" with more experienced nurses. This was called the "buddy system" and was used for students or nurses new to a unit who could benefit from having a nurse familiar with that unit help them in times of need or uncertainty. Being a buddy meant being there for the individual but it did not involve the structure and direction that a preceptorship model would assume.

A mentor is also different from a preceptor in that a mentor is someone who is *selected* by an individual nurse or student nurse and not *assigned* to him or her. A mentor can be someone who does not even work in the same area as the person selecting the mentor. As well, there is a more personal and professional dimension intrinsic to the mentoring role in that the mentor and the person being mentored often stay in touch for many years or actually become close friends.

Being a preceptor, on the other hand, means working with students on a one-to-one basis while they learn how to become professional nurses. Unlike the buddy or mentor experience, the preceptorship experience is a structured one in which you work with a student throughout the teaching/learning process according to specific guidelines, that is, learning/program objectives that provide the parameters around which the preceptorship experience is to be shaped.

Do I have to be a preceptor?

Again, that depends on the area or agency in which you are employed. It may be a requirement or part of your job description to assume the role of preceptor for a certain period of time, and if so it is to your advantage to do so. There is no question, however, that your role as a registered nurse in clinical or community practice is primarily to provide competent and safe care of your assigned patients. Preceptoring is clearly secondary.

What do I get in return for being a preceptor?

That depends. Some programs that offer preceptorship experiences provide preceptors with a letter of commendation from the Dean of the Faculty of Nursing or the Director of Nursing acknowledging their contribution to student learning or the orientation of new nursing staff. In some cases, preceptors are provided with nametags that indicate their status as a preceptor. Others are provided with options to enroll in a variety of university or college courses that are tuition free. And, some preceptors may receive a monetary remuneration for their role. Inevitably, however, it is well documented that nurses who participate as preceptors describe their experiences as extremely rewarding. Remarkably they find that not only do they contribute to student learning but that their learning is increased as well. On a broader perspective, in participating in the preceptorship model of clinical or community teaching you contribute to strengthening the connection between clinical or community practice and education, a connection that is critical to the advancement of the profession of nursing as a whole.

Will I get feedback on my preceptoring behaviors?

This is an area that is important to your professional development. Especially after your first preceptorship experience you will want and need feedback about your preceptoring skills. Feedback with regard to how you are doing as a preceptor may be derived from informally asking others who are in a position to observe you in the preceptor role. Such individuals can include the preceptee, other staff, management, and the faculty contact person. Some programs have a formal evaluation form. The preceptee uses this form to evaluate the preceptor and the results are shared with the preceptor. The value of such a form is that it acknowledges the importance of the preceptor role; assists the preceptee in reflecting upon how the preceptor is performing; and may lead into discussions about evaluation.

What if my preceptee is ill or does not notify me that he or she will not be at work?

Preceptees are being socialized into a professional role. As such they are responsible for notifying you of any absence regardless of the reasons. If a preceptee is ill for a number of days you may have to ask him or her to extend his or her time with you. Preceptees are required to fulfill the mandate of the preceptorship program, and while some may miss a few days throughout the experience and still meet the required time frame, others may be required to extend the time of preceptorship owing to time missed. If the preceptee is from a nursing program, you should notify the faculty contact person. Often, you will find that there are instances during which a student will be ill one day, return for a few days, and then report in ill again. If you observe this pattern of behavior, it is important that you document the days missed and share your findings with the preceptee. Some preceptees may have ongoing health problems that may hinder their progress. They are under no obligation to disclose the specifics of the health problem to you. An alternative placement may have to be arranged, however, or other arrangements pursued so that they are afforded the opportunity to achieve their learning objectives.

What happens if I am ill or unable to continue with the preceptorship experience?

This situation does occur on a fairly regular basis. You may be ill, require an unanticipated leave of absence, or even obtain a new position. If you know in advance that you will be away from the unit, it is important that you arrange for a co-preceptorship with another staff member. In the case of unanticipated illness, and depending on the clinical area, a preceptee may be informed that he or she cannot practice without the preceptor and be subsequently asked to leave. Management personnel may ask another staff member to preceptor or a faculty member may arrange an alternate experience. Not infrequently there have been instances in which preceptors have reported to work despite feeling ill because they knew that a preceptee was relying on them. It is important to remember that precepting is an experience that can and should be shared.

Sample Learning Objectives

Following are sample learning objectives that will provide you with some insights into the expectations often required of undergraduate nursing students in the preceptorship experience. It is important to keep in mind that such learning objectives will vary according to a variety of factors. These include the program of study, the level (year) of the students or where they are in their nursing program, the expectations of the preceptor, and the learning or practice environment.

Following the preceptorship experience, the student will be able to:

Use various forms of knowledge (scientific, personal, aesthetic, ethical) and critical thinking in providing nursing care by:

- Using appropriate resources in collecting data
- Using interviewing skills, observations, and health assessment to collect data
- Systematically collecting relevant data about the patient
- Identifying the patient's stage of growth and development
- Identifying appropriate psychosocial theories

- Using appropriate nursing models to identify positive and negative factors that contribute to the care of the patient
- Accurately recording relevant data
- Reporting relevant data in a clear, concise manner
- Interpreting data by relating to scientific knowledge, concepts, and principles
- Identifying actual and potential problems based on interpretation of assessment data
- Demonstrating the ability to be able to organize care

Administer medications appropriately and safely by:

- Providing a written drug card with dosage indications, precautions, and adverse effects of the patient's prescribed medications
- Relating prescribed medications to the patient's physiological status
- Calculating medication dosage accurately
- Demonstrating the 5 Rs when preparing medications
- Checking intravenous solution
- Determining if intravenous fluid is nearly infused, infiltrated, or stopped
- Regulating intravenous infusion rate accurately
- Changing intravenous solution bag appropriately

Apply nursing care principles in providing patient safety by:

- Identifying and when the physical environment is unsafe for the patient
- Reporting when the physical environment is unsafe for the patient
- Using nursing measures to ensure patient safety
- Performing psychomotor skills with manual dexterity
- Maintaining aseptic technique
- Recognizing obvious breaks in technique

Effectively communicate to develop a professional relationship with patients by:

- Using appropriate verbal and nonverbal communication skills to establish, maintain, and terminate a professional relationship with the patient and family

- Focusing on the patient's concerns
- Communicating empathy, genuineness, and warmth when interacting with the patient and family
- Documenting significant aspects of interaction with the patient and family

Recognize the rights, diversity, and worth of all patients by:

- Facilitating the role of the patient within the health system
- Acknowledging patients' individual beliefs and values
- Respecting patients' rights to privacy, confidentiality, and informed consent
- Identifying potential ethical dilemmas in the practice situation

Collaborate with others in the delivery of health care by:

- Demonstrating a willingness to cooperate with peers, faculty, and other members of the nursing team
- Identifying the role of the nurse in the health care team
- Recognizing the role of other members of the health care team
- Sharing relevant information with peers, preceptor, and other members of the health care team

Use evidence-based practice by:

- Identifying research findings that relate to patient care
- Demonstrating the use of pertinent and up-to-date literature and research findings in providing safe, competent nursing care
- Drawing on different forms of knowledge (scientific, personal, ethical, and aesthetic) when providing nursing care
- Questioning assumptions underlying nursing interventions

Assumes responsibility for learning and competency in her or his nursing practice by:

- Applying knowledge of human, biological, psychological, and physiological sciences in planning and providing nursing care
- Reading relevant research literature in area of specialty
- Understanding legal obligations of practice
- Accepting guidance and supervision of the preceptor
- Being accountable for own nursing care in accordance with agency policies

- Being accountable for meeting practice expectations (ie, being punctual, courteous, and professional)
- Evaluating own performance in providing care for assigned patients
- Assessing personal strengths and weaknesses.

Sample Summary of Preceptee's Prior Experience

John Springer (Fourth-year Nursing Student)

PREVIOUS CLINICAL PLACEMENTS

- Six-week rotation, five days a week, eight hours/day on a cardio-vascular surgical unit
- Twelve weeks in maternal and child (two days per week, eight hours/day). Six in maternal and six in pediatrics
- Six weeks in psychiatric–mental health (two days per week, eight hours/day)
- Six weeks in community health (two days per week, eight hours/day)

SKILLS COMPLETED TO DATE

John has mastered various psychomotor skills in the practice setting for which previous clinical instructors have approved him. These include the following:

- Health assessment
- Family and community assessments
- Preoperative/postoperative nursing care
- Regulation of intravenous fluids
- Administration of oral, intradermal, and intramuscular medications
- Wound care; aseptic technique judged to be excellent
- Catheterization
- Catheter care
- Monitoring of urinary output
- Vital signs including basic ECG interpretation
- Recording of nurses' notes independently

PROCESS SKILLS COMPLETED

- Health teaching
- Discharge planning
- Conflict resolution
- Organizing and prioritizing care for a group of patients
- Beginning competencies in case management

COURSES COMPLETED TO DATE

- All first-year level university required courses completed including pharmacology, pathophysiology, and health assessment
- All second-year nursing courses that included maternal–child and psychiatric–mental health
- All third-year nursing courses including acute adult health
- Currently completing community health nursing course

Fostering Critical Thinking: Sample Scenarios & Questions

Scenario 1

Jane is 21 years old. She is admitted to your unit with acute abdominal pain. She has been diagnosed with pelvic inflammatory disease for which she has been prescribed intravenous antibiotic therapy. In assessing Jane you observe that besides being in considerable stress and discomfort because of her pain, she is also badly bruised with cuts and abrasions evident on her face, neck, torso, and legs. Jane has track marks on her arms and neck that are indicative of a chronic drug user. As well, her clothes are unwashed and her appearance is unkempt. Throughout your assessment you also note that Jane is sometimes withdrawn and noncommittal in her responses to the various questions you ask and other times she seems extremely agitated. As you continue to interact with Jane she informs you that she has been living on the streets since the age of 13. You are struck by her situation. You reflect critically upon Jane's situation and ask yourself several questions:

- First and foremost, what assumptions are you making about Jane and her life's circumstances? For example, because she is a homeless person do you automatically assume that she is from a low socioeconomic background with a family who doesn't care about her? If someone cared about her why would she be living on the streets? If Jane was wealthy and used drugs, how would your perceptions of her differ?

- What conclusions are you drawing from your interactions with Jane?

- What additional information do you require to either confirm or refute your assumptions about Jane and her situation?

Scenario 2

Mrs. Brown is an 82-year-old lady who had been admitted to the emergency department with intractable low back pain. Aside from her pain, Mrs. Brown is very alert and oriented to person, place, and time. Indeed, she is an intelligent woman who has been living independently on her own. On the morning of her admission, Mrs. Brown had called her daughter to tell her that she was unable to move very well. When she had been getting out of bed to go to the bathroom she had experienced a sharp sudden pain in her lower back, which she described as excruciating. Subsequently Mrs. Brown had been unable to move. Her daughter had immediately rushed to her mother's house and after assessing her decided she should call an ambulance to bring her to the hospital. Thus Mrs. Brown, accompanied by her daughter, had waited in the emergency department for 8 hours until a bed had become available. On x-ray it was found that Mrs. Brown had sustained a spontaneous fracture of her lumbar one vertebra because of osteoporosis. Mrs. Brown was administered several doses of morphine in the emergency department to control her pain. In the meantime, Mrs. Brown's daughter had to leave her mother for an hour or so to complete a few chores. While her daughter was away, Mrs. Brown was admitted to the unit where she was prescribed bedrest with intravenous analgesic and anticoagulant therapy. The nurse, upon assessment, finds a rather frail-looking 82-year-old woman who seems to be rather disoriented, at times even incoherent. Encountering Mrs. Brown one of the nurses assumes that she is a frail elderly lady who seems to be out of touch with her surroundings. This nurse would best serve Mrs. Brown by reflecting:

- Why does Mrs. Brown seem so disoriented and out of touch with her surroundings? According to her chart she was alert and oriented when she was admitted to the emergency department.

- Could there be something that has contributed to Mrs. Brown's condition since entering the hospital?
- What impact do staff rotations have on providing continuous care?
- What additional information should the nurse acquire to confirm or refute her assessment?

Scenario 3

Thelma is a 24-year-old patient who has been admitted to the burn unit with extensive second- and third-degree burns throughout her body. Thelma is intelligent, articulate, and quite vocal, even aggressive, in what she does and does not want. In particular she challenges many of the procedures that are carried out by her assigned nurses. Subsequently, many of the nurses are not thrilled at being assigned to care for Thelma. While the nurse who has cared for Thelma over the last 3 days completes Thelma's oral care, Thelma looks at her and says, "Will you please take your time with that, it is hurting me like crazy. I don't know why you can't be more sensitive." The nurse complies. She knows that this must be extremely painful for Thelma because the mucous membrane of her mouth has essentially sloughed off as a result of a medication she had been taking. The nurse waits a few minutes, and then asks Thelma if it okay to proceed. Thelma nods in agreement and says, "I suppose so." This particular nurse had offered to be assigned to Thelma. She liked Thelma's spunk in the face of such adversity. Upon reflecting on her situation, this nurse had asked herself the following questions:

- Why is Thelma so resistant to everything the nurses are doing? Could it be her way of taking back some of the control in her life, particularly in this foreign environment? After all, she is a 24-year-old healthy young woman who is used to being active and independent.
- What assumptions am I making about Thelma's behavior; for example, is it a personal attack on me when she lashes out or is it just a reflection of Thelma's frustration and sense of helplessness?
- Why does Thelma's anger bother staff?
- How best can I support Thelma in helping her get through this ordeal?

Scenario 4

Mr. Springer is a 40-year-old man who has been admitted with a diagnosis of a myocardial infarction. Mr. Springer, aside from this hospitalization, has been someone who has led a fairly healthy life over the years. There is, however, heart disease in his family, and thus, he too has been touched by this familial tendency. Mr. Springer is not married. He has a girlfriend who visits him regularly since his admission and he has two older sisters, Janet and Susan, who clearly adore him. They have been extremely attentive to him and constantly seek out the nurses to question everything that is going on with regard to his care. It is evident from their behavior that Janet and Susan are very anxious about their brother's condition. Their mother died when Mr. Springer was only 6 years old. The sisters were 18 and 20 and essentially assumed the mother role. When assessing this situation, upon critical reflection, as a nurse assigned to Mr. Springer, you ask yourself the following questions:

- What assumptions am I making that contribute or detract from Mr. Springer's particular situation?
- Are there any preconceived notions I hold that would jeopardize the care I am required to give; for example, do I think that the sisters should be less involved? Or do I think they need to be reassured by retaining open communication and support by the nurses and the health team?
- How can I best support Mr. Springer and his significant others in this situation?

Scenario 5

Mr. Springer has been transferred to the step-down unit where you and your preceptor are working. You have been assigned to take care of Mr. Springer. Upon report you have been informed that Mr. Springer's condition has stabilized and he will require routine nursing care and the usual protocol for patients who are postmyocardial infarction. Mr. Springer is still attached to an electrocardiogram monitor as a precautionary measure for the next 24 hours. You have completed your morning care, checked Mr. Springer's vital signs, and had him dangle his feet on the side of the bed for fifteen minutes. He now seems to be resting quite comfortably so you proceed to discard the dirty bed linen and go to the kitchen to make him a fresh drink. When you return to his room, you place the fresh drink on the bedside table, straighten out his bedclothes, and check his pulse simultaneously as you observe the monitor. To your dismay you note that Mr. Springer is experiencing ventricular tachycardia. In this situation you must work very quickly, because the consequences are dire. Your immediate response is to question as follows:

- What is it that I need to do right way besides calling my preceptor?
- What will help Mr. Springer ward off any additional danger? I give Mr. Springer a precordial thump that thankfully returns his rhythm to normal sinus until the appropriate medication (lidocaine) can be administered.
- What should I do now? I stay with Mr. Springer until my preceptor arrives. When she does arrive she immediately administers lidocaine intravenously to control the arrhythmia and prevent the lethal rhythm from recurring.
- Is there anything else that we should do? We administer oxygen 5 liters by nasal prongs to help in the oxygenation of Mr. Springer's myocardium. We then immediately transport him to the coronary care unit for closer monitoring.

Sample Direct Observation

Context

Jean is an experienced nurse and preceptor who works on a cardiovascular surgical step-down unit. She has been working with Suzanne, a fourth year nursing student, for approximately four weeks. For the most part the experience has been progressing well. There have been occasions, however, when Jean has observed that Suzanne has been displaying some difficulty when interacting with patients and their families. While Suzanne would be classified as a very bright and competent student from an organizational and skill level, Jean has been questioning her interpersonal skills particularly with regard to patient situations that require some delicacy and sensitivity. It is fair to say that Jean has subsequently been experiencing some concerns or reservations about Suzanne's capabilities from this perspective. Both Jean and Suzanne have discussed this aspect of her role as a nurse on several occasions but Suzanne does not seem to be making the kind of progress that Jean would expect to see at this stage in her development. Jean has worked with numerous other students over the years so she has a strong sense of the kinds of expectations that are required of a student at this stage in her nursing program. Following is an example of Jean's observation of Suzanne.

Observation

It is Thursday morning. Suzanne is assigned to four patients one of whom is Mr. Macy, a 75-year-old gentleman who recently underwent an abdominal aortic aneurysm repair. He had spent a few days in the intensive care unit following his surgery, was doing very well, and was thus transferred to this step-down unit. On the second day on the unit, however, Mr. Macy had a setback. His condition worsened due to a variety of factors and he was returned to the intensive care unit where he remained for a further week until his condition was stabilized enough to be transferred back to the unit. Mr. Macy has been on this unit now for the past few days and for all intents and purposes, while he is progressing in terms of the surgical procedure itself (his aortic aneurysm repair), he is not improving as rapidly as the doctors and nurses would like. The major concern, for example, is his breathing and his oxygenation. Mr. Macy had developed pneumonia when he had been initially transferred from the intensive care unit and his blood gases have been slow to improve despite the fact that, as recently as yesterday his pneumonia on x-ray appears to be clearing. The doctor thus decided late last evening after reviewing the x-ray that Mr. Macy should have an ultrasound to ascertain if there is anything else, more ominous, that could be contributing to the slow recovery of his blood gases.

Mr. Macy has a very close-knit family. His wife and two daughters have been constantly at his bedside throughout his hospitalization. They are very solicitous of their father's well-being. Up until his surgery, Mr. Macy had been an extremely healthy and active individual. The setback that had required him to be sent back to the intensive care unit has been a cause of great stress for the family. At one point during his stay in the intensive care unit the doctors and nurses had discussed a *do not resuscitate* order with the family. This was completely unexpected to them and caused them a great deal of anxiety at the notion of losing their father when they had not anticipated such an occurrence. Since that experience the family tends to become quite apprehensive about any procedure that is carried out for Mr. Macy. In light of these developments, then, it is essential that the nurses be supportive and sensitive to the family's concerns and make every effort to keep the lines of communication open and clear at all times. So this morning when the older daughter Brittany arrives on the unit and is informed by her father that he has been scheduled for a test she becomes quite concerned. At the time, Suzanne was in

Mr. Macy's room preparing him for his ultrasound and Jean was in earshot so she was able to observe Suzanne's interaction with Mr. Macy and his daughter firsthand. Brittany was clearly quite anxious and asked Suzanne what was going on. Following is their interaction:

Brittany: "Is this anything serious?"

Suzanne: "Not really. At least I don't think so."

Brittany: "Can you tell me exactly what he is having done."

Suzanne: "He is just going to have his lungs checked again to see why his blood gases are not improving more quickly."

Brittany: "Do you mean they suspect there is something else going on with him? Something more than the pneumonia?"

Suzanne: "Probably."

Brittany: "What could they be suspecting?"

Suzanne: "Oh, I wouldn't worry about it. It's probably just something minor."

Brittany: "Such as what?"

Suzanne: "It could be anything I guess. It's probably some kind of growth that's not too serious."

Brittany: "Do you think I could talk directly to the doctor to see what he is thinking."

Suzanne: "Well, I don't think he will be around until later this morning. You could probably talk to him then."

Brittany: "Would it be okay for me to be with dad while he is having the test?"

Suzanne: "I think it would be better if you wait here for him. It shouldn't take too long."

Brittany: "I would really prefer to go with him."

Suzanne: "I will be accompanying him so he will have me there with him."

Brittany: "I guess that will be okay."

At this point Jean intervenes to suggest that perhaps it would be okay for Brittany to accompany her father to the ultrasound department. As it turns out, Mr. Macy is discovered to have a pleural effusion which when aspirated results in a swift recovery. Within a matter of a day or two his blood gases have improved and he himself began to improve rapidly to the joy of his family.

Jean's Response

Following her observation Jean takes a moment during her coffee break to jot down her observation as she had witnessed it. This is often referred to as *anecdotal note or recording* and it does not have to be lengthy. It is important to do this so that you retain an accurate account of exactly what it is that you observe. As you will note, it is important that you recount the observation as accurately as possible. Then, it is also important that you follow it up with your own interpretation of the observation. Jean's note went as follows:

ANECDOTAL NOTE/RECORD OF OBSERVATION

Date: Thursday, November 20, 2003

Time: 0930 hours

Student: Suzanne

Location: Mr. Macy's room

This morning I had occasion to observe Suzanne's interaction with Mr. Macy and one of his daughters. In particular I saw directly how Suzanne responded to Mr. Macy's daughter when she was asking about the test (ultrasound) for which her father had been suddenly scheduled. Suzanne responded to the questions that the daughter had. She provided minimal information. Suzanne made no attempt to inform the daughter or Mr. Macy of the precise nature of the procedure, why exactly he was required to have this done, and what the implications would be to Mr. Macy. When Mr. Macy's daughter asked if she could accompany her father to the procedure, Suzanne immediately vetoed the idea.

Interpretation

From what I observed in this interaction, I would have to say that Suzanne was not at all sensitive to Mr. Macy's daughter's anxiety. When the daughter asked questions of Suzanne to try to glean some kind of reassurance, Suzanne essentially ignored the daughter's cues. I would go so far as to say that Suzanne appeared to be rather flippant in her responses. For example, her statement "Oh, I wouldn't worry about it. It's probably just something minor," I would perceive to be quite dismissive and even unprofessional. When the daughter requested that she be permitted to accompany her father to the ultrasound department, Suzanne immediately vetoed her request. I believe this reflects a lack of sensitivity on her part to the daughter's anxiety and quite dismissive.

Sample Anecdotal Recording

If you have a preceptee who has just administered an intramuscular injection for the first time, your observation might read as follows: *Jane gave her first intramuscular injection today. As arranged, Jane and I met in the med room at the allotted time. Before drawing up the medication, Jane washed her hands and assembled the necessary equipment and supplies, including the ampoule containing the required medication, the appropriate size syringe and needle, and the alcohol swabs. Using the five rights, Jane checked her patient's medication card against the label on the ampoule and then proceeded to draw up the medication. Once completed, she then disposed of the soiled supplies, placing the broken ampoule in the special container for broken glass. We then proceeded to the patient's bedside. Jane approached her patient calling him by name, explaining that she would be giving him his injection, and ensuring that he was appropriately positioned and draped. She administered the injection, asking her patient if he was feeling okay, and when he assured her that he was, we returned to the med room to dispose of the used equipment. Jane then charted the medication in the appropriate manner.*

Your interpretation of this observation might read as follows: I was most impressed with Jane's performance in administering her first intramuscular injection today. Although she was clearly nervous, she was nevertheless organized, using appropriate guidelines to prepare the medication and displaying aseptic technique during preparation and when administering the mediation to the patient. I was particularly struck by the fact that for someone of her years and inexperience, she displayed a distinct level of professionalism, control, and great sensitivity to her patient.

Sample Evaluation Form

This evaluation tool is a five-point scale designed to assess the performance of second-year nursing students being preceptored in the practice setting. It is comprised of *major* learning objectives that are subdivided into behavioral objectives or criteria. The *major* objectives reflect both the curriculum and course objectives of the second-year program while the behavioral objectives/criteria indicate whether the student has achieved these objectives.

Levels of Performance (Key)

Excellent (5)

Consistently meets objectives

Consistently demonstrates initiative and expected level of knowledge in meeting objectives

Rarely requires preceptor assistance

Above Satisfactory (4)	Frequently meets objectives
	Frequently demonstrates initiative and expected level of knowledge in meeting objectives
	Requires preceptor assistance when appropriate
Satisfactory (3)	Usually meets objectives
	Usually demonstrates initiative and expected level of knowledge in meeting objectives
	Requires preceptor assistance when appropriate
Marginal (2)	Frequently fails to meet objectives
	Demonstrates lack of initiative and expected level of knowledge in meeting objectives
	Consistently requires preceptor assistance
Unsatisfactory (1)	Usually fails to meet objectives
	Rarely demonstrates initiative and expected level of knowledge in meeting objectives
	Consistently requires preceptor assistance
Not Observed (No Score)	Objective can be achieved appropriately in the practice setting but is not observed
Not Applicable (No Score)	Objective cannot possibly appropriately be achieved in the practice setting

Definition of Terms

Consistent	Always adheres to the same practice
Inconsistent	Does not always adhere to the same practice
Frequent	Repeatedly occurring
Occasional	Occurring at irregular intervals
Usual	Occurring at regular intervals
Rare	Seldom occurring

Initiative	The ability to think and act independently of another's influence, direction, or suggestion
Expected level of knowledge	Concepts, knowledge, and principles presented to the student to date in nursing and support courses, lectures, laboratories, assigned/suggested readings, and discussion groups
Quality	The degree to which the objective is achieved

A statement(s) by the preceptor will be required in the *Comments* column that will address the quality to which the student achieves the objective.

Guidelines for Use

- This tool is to be completed by the student midway (formative evaluation) into the preceptorship experience and again at the termination of the experience (summative evaluation).

- The tool is to be completed by the preceptor midway into the preceptorship experience and again at the termination of the experience.

- The student will place the appropriate number from the key next to each individual objective.

- The preceptor will place the appropriate number from the key next to each individual objective.

- No numerical score assigned to objectives is Not Observed and Not Applicable.

- The midway evaluation will provide feedback to the student and the preceptor regarding student performance to that date. No grading is assigned at this time.

- The final or summative evaluation is to be completed by the preceptor at the termination of the experience.

- Faculty will grade the final evaluation at the termination of the preceptorship experience with input from the preceptor. This final evaluation will be retained in the student's file.

Calculating the Evaluation Score

The numerical values for the levels of performance (key) range from 5 to 1 with excellent being equal to 5.

To prevent a student's score from being lowered because the practice setting to which he or she is assigned does not permit/require the performance of all of the behavioral objectives, the following formula will be used to calculate the student's score (only observed objectives are included in the score):

$$\frac{\text{Sum of the Scores in Observed Objectives}}{\text{Total Score of the Observed Objectives}} \times \text{Weight} = \text{Mark}$$

For a student to achieve a passing mark, he or she must be observed in a minimum of 46 objectives, as follows:

Uses various forms of knowledge (scientific, personal, aesthetic, ethical) and critical thinking in providing nursing care by:

- Using appropriate resources in collecting data
- Using interviewing skills, observations, and physical assessment to collect data
- Systematically collecting relevant data about the patient
- Identifying the patient's stage of growth and development
- Using a nursing model with which to identify positive and negative factors that contribute to the care of the patient
- Accurately recording relevant data
- Reporting relevant data in a clear, concise manner
- Interpreting data by relating to scientific knowledge, concepts, and principles
- Identifying actual and potential problems based on interpretation of assessment data
- Demonstrating the ability to be able to organize care
- Formulating objectives for patient care
- Providing appropriate rationale for nursing actions
- Identifying relevant nursing interventions
- Adequately preparing patient for nursing interventions
- Identifying the patient's support systems (family, significant other, friends)
- Recognizing the impact that hospitalization has on the patient and family
- Organizing equipment and environment prior to carrying out nursing care
- Providing nursing care in an organized manner
- Setting appropriate priorities when providing care

- Carrying out nursing interventions according to priority
- Providing for patient safety during nursing interventions
- Providing for patient comfort during nursing interventions

Correctly administers medications by:

- Providing a written drug care with dosage indications, precautions, and adverse effects of the patient's prescribed medications
- Relating prescribed medications to the patient's physiological status
- Correctly calculating dosage of medications
- Demonstrating the 5 Rs when preparing medications
- Administering medications appropriately and safely
- Checking if intravenous solution is correct
- Determining if intravenous fluid is nearly infused, infiltrated, or stopped
- Regulating intravenous infusion rate accurately
- Changing intravenous solution bag appropriately

Applies nursing care principles integral to ensuring patient safety by:

- Identifying when the physical environment is unsafe for the patient
- Reporting when the physical environment is unsafe
- Using nursing measures to ensure patient safety
- Performing psychomotor skills with manual dexterity
- Maintaining aseptic technique
- Recognizing obvious breaks in technique

Takes the nutritional status of the patient into account when providing nursing care by:

- Identifying factors that influence the patient's dietary patterns and nutritional status (food preferences, cultural/religious values, psychological variables, personal habits, and physical status)
- Recognizing major factors that contribute to fluid and electrolyte imbalance
- Correctly determining the dietary regimen of the patient
- Relating the patient's regimen to the physiological status
- Accurately recording dietary intake

Completes physical assessment when providing nursing care by:

- Preparing the environment prior to carrying out physical assessment (adjusts lighting, pulls screens/closes door to ensure privacy)
- Ensuring proper positioning of the patient during the assessment
- Using physical assessment skills during the performance of routine nursing care
- Conducting physical assessment in an organized and appropriate manner
- Reporting findings appropriately
- Recording findings accurately

Evaluates nursing care by:

- Determining the actual outcomes of nursing actions
- Comparing actual outcomes of nursing actions with expected outcomes
- Determining the effectiveness of specific interventions
- Identifying the need for alternate nursing interventions
- Planning for alternate nursing interventions

Uses effective communication to develop a professional relationship with patients by:

- Using appropriate verbal and nonverbal communication skills to establish, maintain, and terminate a professional relationship with the patient and family
- Focusing on the patient's concerns
- Communicating empathy, genuineness, and warmth when interacting with the patient and family
- Documenting significant aspects of interaction with the patient and family

Recognizes the rights, diversity, and worth of all patients by:

- Facilitating the role of the patient within the health care system
- Acknowledging the patient's individual beliefs and values
- Respecting the patient's right to privacy, confidentiality, and informed consent
- Identifying potential ethical dilemmas in the practice situation

Collaborates with others in the delivery of health care by:

- Demonstrating a willingness to cooperate with peers, faculty, and other members of the nursing team

- Identifying the role of the nurse in the health care team
- Recognizing the role of other members of the health care team
- Sharing relevant information with peers, preceptor, and other members of the health team

Uses evidence-based practice by:

- Identifying research findings that relate to patient care
- Demonstrating the use of pertinent and up-to-date literature and research findings in providing safe, competent nursing care
- Drawing on different forms of knowledge (scientific, personal, ethical, and aesthetic) when providing nursing care
- Questioning the underlying assumptions of nursing interventions

Demonstrates an awareness of her or his role as a nursing student within the health care team by:

- Determining own specific responsibilities in relation to patients and other team members
- Recognizing that her or his behavior can influence others in the practice setting
- Demonstrating professional behavior while in the practice setting
- Adhering to agency policy regarding dress code
- Demonstrating the ability to work effectively with other members of the nursing team

Assumes responsibility for learning and competency in her or his nursing practice by:

- Applying knowledge of human, biological, psychological, and physiological sciences in planning and providing nursing care
- Accepting guidance and supervision of the preceptor
- Being accountable for own nursing care in accordance with agency policies
- Being accountable for meeting practice expectations
- Evaluating own performance in providing care for assigned patients

Uses knowledge of the change process in the implementation of patient care by:

- Identifying areas requiring improvement in own nursing care
- Promoting planned changes in own behavior through the use of the decision-making process

Five-point Scale Sample Evaluation Form								
Learner Objective	5	4	3	2	1	-	-	Comments
Uses various forms of knowledge and critical thinking by:								
• Uses appropriate resources in collecting data.								
• Uses interviewing skills, observations, physical assessment to collect data.								
• Systematically collects relevant data about the patient.								
• Identifies the patient's stage of growth and development.								
• Uses a nursing model to identify positive and negative factors that contribute to the care of the patient.								
• Accurately records relevant data.								
• Reports relevant data in a clear, concise manner.								
• Interprets data by relating to scientific knowledge, concepts, and principles.								
• Identifies actual and potential problems based on interpretation of assessment data.								
• Demonstrates the ability to be able to organize care.								
• Formulates objectives for patient care.								
• Provides appropriate rationale for nursing actions.								
• Identifies relevant nursing interventions.								
• Adequately prepares patient for nursing interventions.								
• Identifies the patient's support systems (family, significant other, and friends).								
• Recognizes the impact that hospitalization has on the patient and family.								
• Organizes equipment and environment prior to carrying out nursing care.								
• Provides nursing care in an organized manner.								
• Sets appropriate priorities when providing care.								
• Carries out nursing interventions according to priority.								
• Provides for patient safety during nursing interventions.								
• Provides for patient comfort during nursing interventions.								

Pass/Fail Sample Evaluation Form			
Learner Objective	Pass	Fail	Comments
Uses various forms of knowledge and critical thinking by: • Using appropriate resources in collecting data. • Using interviewing skills, observations, and physical assessment to collect data. • Systematically collecting relevant data about the patient. • Identifying the patient's stage of growth and development. • Using a nursing model to identify positive and negative factors that contribute to the care of the patient. • Accurately recording relevant data. • Reporting relevant data in a clear, concise manner. • Interpreting data by relating to scientific knowledge, concepts, and principles. • Identifying actual and potential problems based on interpretation of assessment data. • Demonstrating the ability to be able to organize care. • Formulating objectives for patient care. • Providing appropriate rationale for nursing actions. • Identifying relevant nursing interventions. • Adequately preparing patient for nursing interventions. • Identifying the patient's support systems (family, significant other, and friends). • Recognizing the impact that hospitalization has on the patient and family. • Organizing equipment and environment prior to carrying out nursing care. • Providing nursing care in an organized manner. • Setting appropriate priorities when providing care. • Carrying out nursing interventions according to priority. • Providing for patient safety during nursing interventions. • Providing for patient comfort during nursing interventions.			

Skills Checklist

Name _____   Date _____

Unit _____   Position _____

Preceptor _____   Position _____

Excellent ▼	Satisfactory ▼	Needs Practice ▼	**Handwashing** **Goal:** To prevent and control spread of infection.	**COMMENTS**
___	___	___	1. Stand in front of sink. Do not allow your uniform to touch sink during the washing procedure.	
___	___	___	2. Remove jewelry, if possible, and secure in a safe place or allow plain wedding band to remain in place.	
___	___	___	3. Turn on water and adjust force. Regulate temperature until water is warm.	
___	___	___	4. Wet hands and wrist area. Keep hands lower than elbows to allow water to flow toward fingertips.	
___	___	___	5. Use about 1 teaspoon liquid soap (3–5 mL) from dispenser or rinse bar of soap and lather thoroughly. Cover all areas of hands with soap product. Rinse soap bar again and return to soap dish.	
___	___	___	6. With firm rubbing and circular motions, wash palms and backs of hands, each finger, the areas between fingers, knuckles, wrists, and forearms. Wash at least 1 inch above area of contamination. If hands are not visibly soiled, wash to 1 inch above the wrists.	
___	___	___	7. Continue this friction motion for 10–15 seconds.	
___	___	___	8. Use fingernails of the other hand or a clean orangewood stick to clean under fingernails.	
___	___	___	9. Rinse thoroughly.	
___	___	___	10. Beginning with fingers and moving upward toward forearms, dry hands with a paper towel and discard it immediately. Use another clean towel to turn off faucet. Discard towel immediately without touching other clean hand.	
___	___	___	11. Use lotion on hands if desired.	

Adpated from Taylor, C., Lillis, C., LeMone, P., & LeBon, M. (2001). Procedure checklists to accompany fundamentals of nursing: The art and science of nursing care (4th ed.). Philadelphia: Lippincott Williams & Wilkins.

Sample Verbal Feedback

Situation

It is Thursday morning. Suzanne is assigned to four patients, one of whom is Mr. Macy, a 75-year-old gentleman who recently underwent an abdominal aortic aneurysm repair. He had spent a few days in the intensive care unit following his surgery, was doing very well, and was thus transferred to this step-down unit. On the second day on the unit, however, Mr. Macy had a setback. His condition worsened due to a variety of factors and he was returned to the intensive care unit where he remained for a week until his condition was stabilized enough to be transferred back to the unit. Mr. Macy has been on this unit now for the past few days and for all intents and purposes, though he is progressing in terms of the surgical procedure itself (his aortic aneurysm repair), he is not improving as rapidly as the doctors and nurses would like. The major concern, for example, is his breathing and his oxygenation. Mr. Macy had developed pneumonia when he had been initially transferred from the intensive care unit and his blood gases have been slow to improve despite the fact that as recently as yesterday, his pneumonia, on the x-ray, appeared to be clearing. The doctor thus decided late last evening after reviewing the x-ray that Mr. Macy should have an ultrasound to ascertain if there is anything more ominous that could be contributing to the slow recovery of his blood gases.

Mr. Macy has a very close-knit family. His wife and two daughters have been constantly at his bedside throughout his hospitalization. They are very solicitous of Mr. Macy's well-being. Up until his surgery, Mr. Macy had been an extremely healthy and active individual. The setback that required him to be sent back to the intensive care unit had been a cause of great stress for the family. At one point during his stay in the intensive care unit the doctors and nurses had discussed a *do not resuscitate* order with the family. This was completely unexpected to them and caused them a great deal of anxiety at the notion of losing their father when they had not anticipated such an occurrence. Since that experience the family becomes quite apprehensive about any procedure that is carried out for Mr. Macy. In light of these developments, it is essential that the nurses be supportive and sensitive to the family's concerns and make every effort to keep the lines of communication open and clear at all times. Therefore, this morning when the older daughter Brittany arrives on the unit and is informed by her father that he has been scheduled for a test she becomes quite concerned. At the time, Suzanne was in Mr. Macy's room preparing him for his ultrasound and Jean, Suzanne's preceptor, was in earshot and was able to observe Suzanne's interaction with Mr. Macy and his daughter firsthand. Brittany was clearly quite anxious and asked Suzanne what was going on. Following is their interaction:

Brittany: "Is this anything serious?"

Suzanne: "Not really. At least I don't think so."

Brittany: "Can you tell me exactly what he is having done?"

Suzanne: "He is just going to have his lungs checked again to see why his blood gases are not improving more quickly."

Brittany: "Do you mean they suspect there is something else going on with him? Something more than the pneumonia?"

Suzanne: "Probably."

Brittany: "What could they be suspecting?"

Suzanne: "Oh, I wouldn't worry about it. It's probably just something minor."

Brittany: "Such as what?"

Suzanne: "It could be anything, I guess. It's probably some kind of growth that's not too serious."

Brittany: "Do you think I could talk directly to the doctor to see what he is thinking?"

Suzanne: "Well, I don't think he will be around until later this morning. You could probably talk to him then."

Brittany: "Would it be okay for me to be with Dad while he is having the test?"

Suzanne: "I think it would be better if you wait here for him. It shouldn't take too long."

Brittany: "I would really prefer to go with him."

Suzanne: "I will be accompanying him so he will have me there with him."

Brittany: "I guess that will be okay."

At this point Jean intervenes to suggest that perhaps it would be okay for Brittany to accompany her father to the ultrasound department. As it turns out, Mr. Macy is discovered to have a pleural effusion, which when aspirated results in a swift recovery. Within a matter of a day or two his blood gases have improved and he began to improve rapidly to the joy of his family.

Jean's Verbal Feedback

Following her observation of Suzanne's interaction with Mr. Macy's daughter, Jean takes a moment during her coffee break to jot down some notes about what she had witnessed. It is incumbent on Jean to meet with Suzanne to discuss her observation. Jean makes an appointment with Suzanne to discuss what she has observed and to provide her with some feedback. It will also afford Suzanne an opportunity to respond to Jean's interpretation of the event.

Jean: "So, Suzanne, how do you think you are doing so far?"

Suzanne: "Well, I think everything is going fine. I am really developing some good organizational skills. I am getting lots of experience with dressing changes, IV therapy management, injections, and everything. I am also feeling less nervous about assuming responsibility for the more acute kinds of patients because of my time on this unit."

Jean: "That's good. I am glad to hear that you are becoming more confident in yourself and that you find your time on this unit so rewarding."

Suzanne: "Yes, I think I was so fortunate to have been assigned to this unit. When I talk with my classmates I realize that compared to many of them I am getting so much more experience than they seem to be getting."

Jean: "Suzanne, when you say you are getting more experience, to what exactly are you referring?"

Suzanne: "As I said, dressing changes, IV management, all of those kinds of things."

Jean: "So then, from what you are saying, am I to assume that you think that nursing is mostly about doing dressings, changing IV bags, etc.?"

Suzanne: "I guess I would agree with that."

Jean: "Remember a few weeks ago we discussed how important interpersonal communication is in this role?"

Suzanne: "Yes, I remember."

Jean: "Do you also remember that we had discussed ways in which you could improve your own interpersonal communication skills?"

Suzanne: "Yes, I remember. But to be honest with you, I am not always very comfortable in the different situations that I encounter. I don't always feel very confident when I'm talking to patients and their families."

Jean: "How do you think you did this morning with Mr. Macy and his daughter?"

Suzanne: "I thought I did okay."

Jean: "Do you think you were sensitive to Mr. Macy's daughter?"

Suzanne: "I think so. I answered her questions when she asked."

Jean: "Were you aware how anxious she was?"

Suzanne: "What do you mean?"

Jean: "Well, do you think telling her not to worry about anything was sensitive?"

Suzanne: "I thought I was just being reassuring."

Jean: "But what is your responsibility as a nurse in this situation?"

Suzanne: "To be reassuring."

Jean: "I agree. But don't you need to be aware of all of the facts before you give this kind of reassurance?"

Suzanne: "What do you mean?"

Jean: "Well, Mr. Macy was going for an ultrasound to determine if there was something more serious going on with him. You no doubt read that on his chart—that the doctors were concerned that he might have some kind of underlying malignancy?"

Suzanne: "Yes, I guess I read that. But I didn't want to tell the daughter that because it would upset her even more."

Jean: "Do you think that was appropriate?"

Suzanne: "Now that we talk about it, I guess it wasn't."

Jean: "How do you think you could have handled the situation differently?"

Suzanne: "I guess I could have been more sensitive. I could have talked to her more directly about what was going on with her father but in a way that would not have caused her to be more anxious. I could have explained what an ultrasound is and that it helps to detect anything that may not be evident on an x-ray. I guess I could have been more honest and direct. But to tell you the truth I am not very comfortable or confident with that."

Jean: "So then, how can we work on helping you to become more comfortable and confident in these kinds of situations? What is it that we can do together to help you to improve, because I cannot emphasize enough how important it is for you to communicate well with your patients and their families. That is a big part of what it means to be a nurse."

Suzanne: "Maybe I could watch you more often in dealing with these kinds of situations. I have been so busy focusing on my skills, I guess I neglected this aspect of my performance."

Jean: "Okay, I think that is an excellent solution. Over the next 2 weeks, we will work together in this way. I will have you observe me as to how I interact in these kinds of situations. Then I will have you interact in a similar situation as it arises. We will meet as we are doing today and have a debriefing."

Suzanne: "That sound good. I think that will help me so much. I really want to be a good nurse. I've always wanted to be a nurse."

Jean: "Okay, then, that will be our plan. I also want to say, though, that we need to put a timeline on this. We will work on this aspect of your performance over the next month and meet regularly during that time. If after that month, however, you have still not progressed we will seriously need to consider whether you should pass this rotation. Do you understand that?"

Suzanne: "Yes, I understand."

Jean: "But, Suzanne, if we work together on this, I know you can be successful."

Sample Preceptee Self-Evaluation Form

U sually throughout the preceptorship experience, preceptees arc expected to conduct a self-evaluation. This self-evaluation is based on the evaluation form or rating scale by which the preceptor evaluates them. It is, therefore, critical that preceptees review that evaluation form on a regular basis to ascertain how well they are meeting or achieving the particular objectives delineated in that form. It is also incumbent on preceptees to discuss their progress with their preceptors and to specifically seek out their assistance if they should find that they are not achieving the objectives. In reviewing their own performance, it is prudent for preceptees, in addition to following the evaluation form, to ask the following questions:

- Am I achieving the objectives outlined on this form?
- How would I rate myself on the learning objectives?
- Can I be doing better in achieving the various objectives?

- If I am hesitant or discovering that I am unable to achieve certain objectives, how do I go about improving the potential for meeting them?

- What do I do if it is virtually impossible to meet some of the objectives because of the nature of the unit to which I have been assigned?

Assessing Learning Style: How Do I Learn Best?

Please choose one answer although all answers to the question may be true. It is your first reaction that is important.

1. Your new student needs to go to Human Resources. Since she has not worked in your agency before she does not know where it is. You **initially** would:
a. ___ draw her a map
b. ___ tell her how to get there
c. ___ write down the directions
d. ___ take her down there if you had the time

2. If you were your student, which approach would you have preferred?
a. ___ having a map
b. ___ being told how to get there
c. ___ having written instructions
d. ___ being taken down there

3. You have been asked to teach about advanced nutrition support to a small group of students. In planning how you would do this, you **initially** think of:
a. ___ using diagrams
b. ___ talking to them about back care
c. ___ giving them handouts
d. ___ doing a demonstration

4. You are going to cook a dessert as a special treat. Do you:
a. ___ search cookbooks looking for ideas
b. ___ ask others for good recipes
c. ___ refer to a specific cookbook with good recipes
d. ___ cook something familiar without instructions

5. You are going to purchase a new stereo. Other than price, what would influence you?
a. ___ distinctive, upscale appearance
b. ___ a friend talking about it
c. ___ reading the details about it
d. ___ listening to it

6. You are not sure whether to spell a word as "paediatric" or "pediatric". Do you:
a. ___ see the word in your mind
b. ___ sound it out
c. ___ look it up in the dictionary
d. ___ write both versions down

7. Do you prefer a teacher who likes to use:
a. ___ diagrams and charts
b. ___ discussion methods
c. ___ handouts
d. ___ practical sessions

8. Which of the following games do you prefer?
a. ___ Pictionary
b. ___ Monopoly
c. ___ Scrabble
d. ___ Charades

9. How do you like to spend your leisure time?
a. ___ going to a movie
b. ___ visiting with friends and relatives
c. ___ reading a good novel
d. ___ exercising

10. You are expected to learn a new procedure at work. You would prefer if someone would **initially**:
a. ___ let you see the procedure
b. ___ explain it to you
c. ___ give you a written description
d. ___ demonstrate it

To obtain your score, count the number of a's _____ b's _____ c's _____ d's _____
High score of a's means you are visual, of b's means you are aural, of c's means you prefer reading and writing, and of d's means you are kinesthetic.

Sample Learning Contract

The learning contract is a valuable learning tool for both you and your preceptee. It provides an explicit or concrete picture of what it is you are both expecting regarding the preceptee's performance. Let us look at a specific example. You are working with a beginning student, and you have observed that for the past 2 weeks she is consistently late to the unit and subsequently must seek assistance with getting up to speed. As well, you also observe that she spends little time interacting with her assigned patient. After 2 weeks of voicing your concerns regarding these two particular behaviors to your preceptee, you note that there is no discernible improvement. This is a good time to enter into a learning contract with the preceptee. To that end, it is wise to schedule a meeting at a time during which there will be no interruptions. You discuss again your observations and concerns, seek the preceptee's perspective, and introduce the notion of a learning contract. You indicate to the preceptee that you would like to observe a change in her behavior within a specific time frame. Therefore, you believe it is best to outline both of your expectations and a time frame in which you would like to see improvement. The contract usually comprises six components: the goals and objectives that must be achieved at the termination of the contract, specific learning activities that must be achieved within a specific time period, preceptor/preceptee expectations, method of evaluation, specific timelines, and grading where appropriate (Gaberson & Oermann, 1999). A learning contract resembles the following:

Name of Preceptee:

Name of Preceptor:

Beginning Date of Contract:

Termination Date of Contract:

Name of Relevant Faculty:

Course:

A. Preceptee's specific goals and objectives to be achieved (written by preceptee):

B. Exact learning activities to be carried out by the preceptee to fulfill this learning contract:

C. Preceptor's specific expectations for this contract:

D. Exact time frame (dates and times) in which activities are to be achieved:

E. Evaluation methods: How will this contract be achieved successfully? Set specific criteria.

F. Grade (if appropriate):

G. Agreement. In writing indicate as follows: "This learning contract is binding on the preceptee who agrees with the preceptor that the contract will be fulfilled only when and if the objectives and described learning activities are achieved to the satisfaction of both parties."

H. Signature of Preceptee:

Signature of Preceptor:

Signature of Relevant Faculty:

Date: Time:

Index

Page numbers followed by b indicate box.

Difficult situations, 113–121. *See also*
    Learning opportunities
Diverger learning style, 99
Documentation
    in difficult situations, 120–121
    for evaluation, 91

E

Encouragement, 39–40
Ethical issues, 119–120
Evaluation, 67–68, 142
    by faculty, 53–54, 53b
    formative, 132
    models of, 67
    preceptee self-evaluation, 49–50, 49b,
      93
    by preceptor, 40–42, 41b
    of preceptorship, 139–140
    summative, 132
    techniques for, 90–93
      anecdotal recording, 91
      feedback, 92–93
      observation, 90–91
    tools for, 67, 132
      checklists, 75b, 92
      rating scales, 91–92
    unsatisfactory, 29, 68. *See also* Learn-
      ing opportunities

F

Facilitation
    critical thinking and, 81–82, 81b
    by preceptor, 38–40, 38b
    vs. guidance, 81
Faculty
    as custodian of teaching-learning
      process, 9–10
    involvement of, 9–10, 11b, 12–13
    patient assignments and input of,
      77–78
    role of, 50–55, 143
      custodian, 51–52, 52b
      evaluator, 53–54, 53b
      resource, 50–51, 51b
      role model, 54–55, 54b
Faculty-student ratio, 9
Feedback
    evaluation and, 92–93

giving, 27, 41, 125–127, 133
ongoing, 132
verbal, 126–127
written, 127
Formative evaluation, 132

G

Gift exchanging, 29, 132, 140
Global learners, 102
Goals and objectives for preceptorship,
    39, 57–68, 69b, 139. *See also*
    Learning objectives
    of administration, 60–61
    of educational program, 51–52,
      57–60
    of preceptee, 61–65
    of preceptor, 61–65
Guardian, preceptor as, 42, 42b
Guidance
    critical thinking and, 80, 81b
    by preceptor, 40–41, 40b
    vs. facilitation, 81

H

Hospitable climate, 19b, 20–21

I

Independent study, 87b, 88
Inservices, 87b, 89
Interview, for learning style, 101–102

K

Kinesthetic learning, 101

L

Learning, 97–110
    adult, 19b–20b, 100
    auditory, 100
    cycle of, 99
    dialogue and, 108–109
    modalities of
      auditory, 100
      kinesthetic, 101
      tactile, 100–101
      visual, 100